Detailed Healthy
Slow Cooker

100 Recipes Cokbook

Savor the Flavor: Slow Cooker Recipes for Busy Lives

By Amelia Rose Garcia

TABLE OF CONTENTS

Introduction to Slow Cooking

Slow cooking is a traditional cooking method that has gained popularity in contemporary kitchens because of its ease of use, capacity to soften tough meat cuts, and flavor-enhancing properties. The method involves cooking food at a low temperature over an extended period, typically in a slow cooker, an electrical appliance designed for this purpose. This introduction explores the history, benefits, techniques, and diverse culinary applications of slow cooking.

History and Evolution of Slow Cooking

Slow cooking can trace its roots back to ancient civilizations where cooking over a low fire or in clay pots was common. Cultures worldwide have versions of slow-cooked dishes, such as stews, braises, and roasts. The modern slow cooker, also known as a Crock-Pot, was invented in the early 1970s by Irving Naxon. He was inspired by his Jewish grandmother's method of making cholent, a traditional Sabbath stew. This invention revolutionized home cooking, allowing busy families to prepare meals conveniently and efficiently.

The Science Behind Slow Cooking

The science of slow cooking is centered on heat transfer and moisture retention principles. Slow cookers operate at temperatures ranging from 170°F (77°C) to 280°F (138°C). This low-temperature cooking allows for the gradual breakdown of connective tissues and collagen in meats, resulting in tender and flavorful dishes. The sealed environment of a slow cooker also minimizes moisture loss, ensuring that food remains moist and infused with its juices and the flavors of added ingredients.

Benefits of Slow Cooking

Convenience

Convenience is one of the main advantages of slow cooking.
The slow cooker takes little attention once ingredients are prepa red and added, so you can spend more time on other things.
This is particularly helpful for people who work or have busy fa milies.

Flavor Enhancement

Slow cooking allows tastes to meld and intensify, creating richer, more complex flavors.
The meal's flavor profile is improved by the lengthy infusion of s pices, herbs, and aromatics.

Nutritional Retention

Slow cooking often retains more nutrients than other cooking methods, such as boiling or frying. The low and steady heat helps preserve vitamins and minerals that might otherwise be lost through high-temperature cooking.

Cost-Effectiveness

By utilizing cheaper cuts of meat that benefit from slow cooking's tenderizing effect, delicious meals can be created on a budget. Additionally, slow cookers are energy-efficient, using less electricity than conventional ovens.

Slow Cooking Techniques

Preparation

Practical slow cooking starts with proper preparation. This involves selecting the right ingredients, cutting vegetables and meats into uniform sizes for even cooking, and considering the layering of ingredients within the slow cooker. Denser items like root vegetables are typically placed at the bottom, while more delicate ingredients are added later in the cooking process.

Browning

Browning meats and veggies before putting them in the slow coo ker can greatly improve flavor, though it's not always necessary. The Maillard reaction adds a savory, rich flavor that enhances th e dish's overall flavor character.

Layering

The order in which ingredients are layered in the slow cooker can impact the cooking process. Denser vegetables should be placed at the bottom, followed by meats and lighter vegetables or grains. This ensures even cooking and prevents delicate ingredients from becoming mushy.

Timing

Cooking times vary depending on the ingredients.
To get the right texture and flavor, it's important to know how lo ng certain ingredients should cook for.For instance, tougher cuts of meat may require 8-10 hours of cooking on low, whereas more delicate vegetables might only need a few hours.

Liquid Management

Slow cookers typically require less liquid than traditional cooking methods because they retain moisture well. Adjusting the amount of liquid in recipes is essential to avoid overly watery dishes. Sauces and broths should be used sparingly, and thicker liquids can be added towards the end of the cooking process.

Types of Slow Cookers

Basic Slow Cookers

The most common type of slow cooker features a simple ceramic or metal pot encased in a heating element. These models often have basic settings such as low, high, and warm and are ideal for straightforward slow-cooking tasks.

Programmable Slow Cookers

More advanced models come with programmable settings that allow users to set precise cooking times and temperatures. These slow cookers often include features like delayed start, automatic switch to warm mode, and digital displays.

Multi-Function Cookers

Modern kitchen appliances, such as the Instant Pot, combine the functionalities of a slow cooker, pressure cooker, rice cooker, and more. These multi-function cookers offer versatility and can streamline meal preparation.

Culinary Applications of Slow Cooking

Soups and Stews

Slow cookers are particularly well-suited for making soups and stews, where the extended cooking time allows flavors to meld beautifully. Classic examples include beef stew, chicken noodle soup, and vegetable chili.

Braises

Braising tough cuts of meat in a slow cooker yields tender, flavorful results. Dishes like pot roast, coq au vin, and pulled pork benefit from the low and slow cooking, breaking down connective tissues and infusing the meat with flavor.

Beans and Legumes

Slow cooking is ideal for preparing beans and legumes, which require long cooking times to become tender. Chili, lentil soup, and baked beans are perfect for slow cookers.

Desserts

Desserts like cheesecakes, cobblers, and bread pudding can all b e prepared in slow cookers. The gentle, even heat ensures desserts cook thoroughly without burning or drying out.

Cultural Perspectives on Slow Cooking

Different cultures have embraced slow cooking in various forms, each with unique recipes and techniques. Understanding these cultural perspectives enriches our appreciation of slow cooking as a global culinary practice.

French Cuisine

In French cuisine, slow cooking is epitomized by boeuf bourguignon and cassoulet. These hearty dishes use robust ingredients and long cooking times to develop deep, complex flavors.

Asian Cuisine

Asian cuisines also feature slow-cooked dishes, such as Chinese red-cooked pork and Japanese nikujaga. These dishes often balance sweet, savory, and umami flavors, with ingredients simmered over low heat to achieve tenderness and flavor integration.

Latin American Cuisine

Latin American dishes like Mexican barbacoa and Brazilian feijoada showcase slow cooking techniques. These dishes often utilize bold spices and seasonings, with slow cooking ensuring that flavors penetrate the ingredients thoroughly.

Tips for Successful Slow Cooking

Plan Ahead

Practical slow cooking requires planning. Select recipes that fit your schedule, prepare ingredients in advance, and ensure you have enough cooking time to achieve the desired results.

Use Fresh Ingredients

Fresh, high-quality ingredients enhance the flavor and texture of slow-cooked dishes. Avoid over-relying on processed or canned ingredients, which can compromise the dish's taste.

Avoid Overfilling

Overfilling the slow cooker can lead to uneven cooking and spillage. To allow for proper heat circulation, it is recommended that the slow cooker be filled no more than two-thirds to three-quarters full.

Monitor Consistency

Periodically check the consistency of your dish, especially towards the end of the cooking time. Adjust seasoning, add liquid if necessary, and ensure ingredients are cooked to your preference.

Common Challenges and Solutions in Slow Cooking

Overcooking

Overcooking is a common issue with slow cooking, particularly for delicate ingredients. To prevent this, adhere to recommended cooking times and consider using advanced slow cookers' programmable features.

Bland Flavors

Slow-cooked dishes can sometimes need more intensity of flavor. To counter this, season generously, use robust ingredients, and consider browning meats and vegetables beforehand.

Soggy Vegetables

Vegetables can become overly soft in a slow cooker. To avoid this, add vegetables later in the cooking process or cut them into larger pieces to maintain texture.

Conclusion

Slow cooking is a versatile and valuable technique in the culinary world, offering numerous benefits, including convenience, flavor enhancement, nutritional retention, and cost-effectiveness. Understanding the principles and methods of slow cooking can elevate everyday meals, making it easier to prepare delicious, wholesome dishes with minimal effort. By embracing the rich traditions and modern innovations of slow cooking, home cooks can enjoy the satisfaction of creating flavorful, tender, and nutritious meals for themselves and their loved ones.

SLOW COOKER 100 RECIPES COKBOOK:RECIPES

INGREDIENTS

- ❖ 2 pounds beef stew meat and cut into 1-inch cubes
- ❖ 1/4 cup all-purpose flour
- ❖ 1/2 teaspoon salt
- ❖ 1/2 teaspoon black pepper
- ❖ 2 tablespoons olive oil (optional for browning)
- ❖ 1 clove garlic, minced
- ❖ 1 bay leaf
- ❖ 1 teaspoon paprika
- ❖ 1 teaspoon Worcestershire sauce
- ❖ 1 large onion, chopped
- ❖ 1 1/2 cups beef broth
- ❖ 3 large potatoes, peeled and diced
- ❖ 4 carrots, peeled and sliced
- ❖ 2 stalks celery, sliced

INSTRUCTIONS

Gather ingredients:

1. Mix flour, pepper, and salt in a big plastic bag. Stir in meat cubes after coating.
2. Chop celery, carrots, potatoes, and onion.
3. Optional meat browning: Cook olive oil in a skillet over medium-high heat. After adding the beef cubes, brown them all over. This step adds flavor to the stew but is optional.
4. Add to slow cooker: Place meat in slow cooker bottom.

5. Combine diced onion, paprika, bay leaf, Worcestershire sauce, and garlic.
6. Mix in beef stock.
7. Layer celery, carrots, and potatoes over the meat and season.

Chef:

1. Cover and simmer on Low for 8–10 hours or High for 4–6 hours when the meat and veggies are soft.
2. Serve the stew after tasting and adjusting spices.
3. Take out the bay leaf.
4. Serve hot with mashed potatoes or crusty toast.

NOTE:

➢ Browning beef cubes before slow cooking enhances stew flavor.
➢ Turnips and parsnips can be added or removed.
➢ To make the stew more luscious, add 2 teaspoons cornstarch and 2 tablespoons water. Cook on high for 30 minutes.
➢ Leftover stew can be frozen for three months or refrigerated for three days in an airtight container. Can you heat it well before serving?

2. SLOW COOKER CHICKEN AND DUMPLINGS

INGREDIENTS

- ❖ 4 boneless, skinless chicken breasts
- ❖ 1 onion, finely chopped
- ❖ 2 cups chicken broth
- ❖ 2 cans (10.5 ounces each) cream of chicken soup
- ❖ 1 teaspoon dried thyme
- ❖ 1 teaspoon dried parsley
- ❖ Salt and pepper to taste
- ❖ 4 large carrots, sliced
- ❖ 2 stalks celery, sliced
- ❖ 1 cup frozen peas
- ❖ 1 can (16.3 ounces) refrigerated biscuit dough, cut into quarters

INSTRUCTIONS

1. Fill the slow cooker with chicken breasts, laying them on the bottom.
2. Add chicken broth, cream of chicken soup, diced onion, parsley, thyme, salt, and pepper.
3. Include celery and carrots.
4. Cover and stew the chicken for 6–8 hours on low or 3–4 hours on high until tender and done.

To shred chicken

1. remove the breasts and shred them with two forks an hour before serving.
2. Place the chicken shreds back into the slow cooker.

Include Dumplings:

1. Add the frozen peas and stir.
2. Place the quarters of biscuit dough on top of the chicken mixture.

Make dumplings:

1. Cook the dumplings on High, covered, for 30 to 1 hour or until they are fluffy and well-cooked.

Serve:

➤ Provide hot food.

NOTE:

➤ Sear chicken breasts in a skillet before adding to the slow cooker for flavor.
➤ Feel free to add extra veggies, such as maize or green beans.
➤ You can keep leftover chicken and dumplings in the fridge for up to three days if you store them in an airtight container.

2. SLOW COOKER PORK CARNITAS

INGREDIENTS

- ❖ 4 pounds pork shoulder and cut into large chunks
- ❖ 1 tablespoon salt
- ❖ 1 teaspoon black pepper
- ❖ 1 tablespoon ground cumin
- ❖ 1 tablespoon dried oregano
- ❖ 1 onion, chopped
- ❖ 4 cloves garlic, minced
- ❖ 2 jalapeños, chopped
- ❖ 1 orange, cut in half
- ❖ 1/2 cup chicken broth

INSTRUCTIONS

Get the ingredients ready:

1. Combine the oregano, cumin, salt, and pepper in a small bowl.
2. Spread the spice mixture evenly over the slices of pork shoulder.
3. Include in the Slow Cooker:
4. The pork should be put in the slow cooker.
5. Add the chopped jalapeños, garlic, and onion.
6. After adding the orange halves to the slow cooker, squeeze the juice over the meat.
7. Add the chicken broth.

Cook:

1. Cover the pork and cook on Low for 8–10 hours or High for 4–6 hours until fork-tender.

Crisp and Shred Pork:

2. Preheat oven to high broil.
3. Two forks remove and shred pork from slow cooker.
4. Pour cooking juice over pork shreds on a baking sheet.
5. Broil pork for five minutes to crisp the edges.
6. Serve pork carnitas on warm tortillas with chopped onions, salsa, lime wedges, and cilantro.

NOTE:

➢ Crisping the pork under the broiler gives carnitas a great texture, but it's optional.
➢ Leftover carnitas can be frozen for three months or refrigerated for three days in an airtight container.

4. COOKER VEGETARIAN CHILI

INGREDIENTS

- ❖ 1 onion, chopped
- ❖ 3 cloves garlic, minced
- ❖ 1 bell pepper, chopped
- ❖ 1 zucchini, chopped
- ❖ 2 carrots, sliced
- ❖ 1-can (15-ounce) drained, washed black beans
- ❖ 1 can (15 ounces) drained, washed kidney beans
- ❖ 1 can (15 ounces) pinto beans, drained and rinsed
- ❖ 1 can (28 ounces) diced tomatoes
- ❖ 1 can (6 ounces) tomato paste
- ❖ 2 cups vegetable broth
- ❖ 1 tablespoon chili powder
- ❖ 1 teaspoon ground cumin
- ❖ 1 teaspoon paprika
- ❖ 1/2 teaspoon cayenne pepper (optional)
- ❖ Salt and pepper to taste

INSTRUCTIONS

Add to Slow Cooker:

1. Fill the slow cooker with the diced carrots, bell pepper, onion, and zucchini.
2. Incorporate the diced tomatoes, kidney beans, pinto beans, black beans, tomato paste, and vegetable broth.
3. Add the chili powder, cumin, paprika, salt, pepper, and cayenne (if using).

Chef:

1. After the vegetables are soft, cover and simmer on Low for 6 to 8 hours or on High for 3 to 4 hours.
2. Serve: The chili can be served hot with avocado slices, sour cream, chopped green onions, or shredded cheese on top if preferred.

NOTES:

➢ This chili can be used for many purposes. You are welcome to add spinach, corn, or mushrooms, among other vegetables.
➢ You can add one cup of cooked quinoa or one cup of cooked bulgur wheat for extra protein.
➢ Chili leftovers can be refrigerated for up to three days in an airtight container or frozen for up to three months.

5. SLOW COOKER LAMB SHANKS

INGREDIENTS

- ❖ 4 lamb shanks
- ❖ Salt and pepper to taste
- ❖ 2 tablespoons olive oil
- ❖ 1 onion, chopped
- ❖ 3 cloves garlic, minced
- ❖ 2 carrots, chopped
- ❖ 2 stalks celery, chopped
- ❖ 1 can (14.5 ounces) diced tomatoes
- ❖ 1 cup red wine
- ❖ 1 cup beef broth
- ❖ 1 teaspoon dried rosemary
- ❖ 1 teaspoon dried thyme
- ❖ 2 bay leaves
- ❖ 1 tablespoon tomato paste
- ❖ 1 teaspoon Worcestershire sauce (optional)
- ❖ Fresh parsley, chopped (for garnish)

INSTRUCTIONS

1. Prepare the ingredients by liberally seasoning the lamb shanks with salt and pepper.
2. Over medium-high heat, brown lamb shanks in olive oil in a large skillet. While adding lamb shanks, sear for four to five minutes. After browning lamb shanks, simmer them.
3. Sauté chopped onion, celery, carrots, and garlic in the same skillet. Simmer for five minutes to tenderize vegetables. After sautéing, add vegetables to slow cooker.

Include the Remaining Contents:

1. Fill the slow cooker with the diced tomatoes, red wine, beef broth, bay leaves, thyme, rosemary, and Worcestershire sauce (if using). Mix well to blend.Simmer:
2. Cover and boil lamb shanks on Low for 8–10 hours or High for 4
3. –6 hours until tender and falling off the bone.
4. Final step: remove the slow cooker bay leaves.
5. After tasting
6. , salt and pepper the Sauce.

NOTE

1. Lamb shanks should be deep brown before simmering to bring out their rich flavor. This step is recommended for best results
2. , but you can skip it.
3. Instead of red wine, use beef broth or an alcohol-free red wine replacement.
4. Variations of vegetables: Slow cookers taste and feel better with parsnips and mushrooms.
5. For a more tasty sauce, Mix one tablespoon cornstarch and two teaspoons water and add to the slow cooker 30 minutes before cooking. Slow-cook sauce until thick.
6. Storage: Chilled lamb shanks can be kept in the refrigerator for up to three days or frozen for up to three months when kept in an airtight container. Before serving, could you give them a thorough heat?
7. Savor your tender and tasty lamb shanks that are slow-cooked to perfection!

6. SLOW COOKER POT ROAST

INGREDIENTS

- ❖ Three to four pounds of roast beef chuck
- ❖ To taste, add salt and pepper.
- ❖ Two tsp olive oil
- ❖ one sliced onion
- ❖ three minced garlic cloves
- ❖ four big carrots that have been peeled and sliced
- ❖ 4 big potatoes, chopped into bits after peeling
- ❖ 2 stalks celery, cut into chunks
- ❖ 1 cup beef broth
- ❖ 1 cup red wine (optional; can substitute with additional beef broth)
- ❖ 2 tablespoons tomato paste
- ❖ 1 tablespoon Worcestershire sauce
- ❖ 1 teaspoon dried thyme
- ❖ 1 teaspoon dried rosemary
- ❖ 2 bay leaves
- ❖ Fresh parsley, chopped (for garnish)

INSTRUCTIONS

Get the ingredients ready:

1. Give the beef chuck roast a liberal amount of salt and pepper.
2. Place a large skillet over medium-high heat with olive oil to brown the roast. After adding the beef chuck roast, cook it on each side for 4–5 minutes. After it has browned, place the roast in the slow cooker.

Sauté Vegetables:

1. Chop onion and garlic and add to skillet. Simmer onion for 3–4 minutes to tenderize. Stir sautéed garlic and onion into the slow cooker.
2. Slow cooker vegetables and liquid: Add carrots, potatoes, and celery
3. to the roast.
4. Add tomato paste, Worcestershire sauce, thyme, rosemary, red wine (if used), and beef broth to a bowl. Cover the slow cooker roast and veggies with the mixture.
5. Use bay leaves.
6. Simmer covered for 8–10 hours on Low or 4–6 hours on High until veggies are cooked and roast is mushy.
7. Before serving, close the slow cooker and remove bay leaves.
8. Add salt and pepper to taste.
9. Slicing or shredding
10. the pot roast, serve it hot with vegetables and sauce. Sprinkle fresh parsley.

NOTE:

➤ Browning beef chuck roast before slow cooking adds flavor.Recommended for optimum outcomes, but optional.
➤ Beef broth or non-alcoholic red wine can replace red wine.
➤ Vegetables Parsnips, turnips, and mushrooms add flavor and texture to slow cookers.
➤ Add one tablespoon cornstarch and two teaspoons water 30 minutes before cooking to thicken the slow cooker sauce. Tighten sauce by overcooking.

➢ A tightly sealed pot roast can be frozen for three months or refrigerated for three days. It should be warmed fully before serving.
➢ Your classic pot roast is always appropriate!

7. SLOW COOKER LENTIL SOUP

INGREDIENTS

- ❖ 2 cups dried lentils, rinsed and sorted
- ❖ 1 onion, chopped
- ❖ 3 cloves garlic, minced
- ❖ 3 carrots, peeled and chopped
- ❖ 3 celery stalks, chopped
- ❖ 1 can (14.5 ounces) diced tomatoes
- ❖ 6 cups vegetable broth
- ❖ 1 teaspoon dried thyme
- ❖ 1 teaspoon dried oregano
- ❖ 1 teaspoon ground cumin
- ❖ 1/2 teaspoon smoked paprika (optional)
- ❖ Salt and pepper to taste
- ❖ 2 bay leaves
- ❖ 2 cups spinach or kale, chopped (optional)
- ❖ 1 tablespoon lemon juice (optional for brightness)
- ❖ Fresh parsley, chopped (for garnish)

INSTRUCTIONS

Get the ingredients ready:

1. After rinsing, remove any small stones or dirt from the lentils.
2. Chop the celery, carrots, onion, and garlic.

Include in the Slow Cooker:

1. Add the diced tomatoes, chopped onion, celery, carrots, and garlic to the slow cooker and the rinsed lentils.

2. Add the broth made of vegetables.
3. Add the bay leaves, salt, pepper, thyme, oregano, cumin, and smoked paprika.

Cook:

1. The lentils and veggies should be soft after 6–8 hours on Low or 3–4 hours on High.
2. In the last 30 minutes of cooking, add chopped kale or spinach to finish the soup.
3. For added brightness, stir in the lemon juice shortly before serving.

Take out the bay leaf.

➤ Serve the hot lentil soup with freshly chopped parsley on top. It goes nicely with a side salad or crusty bread.

NOTE

Lentil Varieties:

1. Red, brown, or green lentils work well in this soup. Remember that red lentils have a thicker consistency and cook more rapidly before becoming mushy.

Taste Differences:

1. For more flavor, stir in a teaspoon of tomato paste, or add a dash of red pepper flakes for some heat.

Boost Your Protein

1. : During the last hour of cooking, simmer a can of rinsed and drained white beans or chickpeas to provide even more protein.

Storage:

1. Leftover lentil soup can be frozen for up to three months or refrigerated for up to five days if stored in an airtight container. Reheat through well before serving.

Thickness Adjustment:

1. Add extra water or vegetable broth to ensure consistency if the soup is too thick.
2. Enjoy this hearty and nutritious slow-cooked lentil soup!

INGREDIENTS

- ❖ 6 slices bacon, chopped
- ❖ Three pounds of 1-inch-cube-sized beef chuck roast
- ❖ Salt and pepper to taste
- ❖ 1 cup pearl onions (frozen or fresh, peeled)
- ❖ 4 cloves garlic, minced
- ❖ 2 carrots, sliced
- ❖ 2 stalks celery, chopped
- ❖ 1 pound mushrooms, sliced
- ❖ 2 tablespoons tomato paste
- ❖ 2 cups red wine (preferably Burgundy or Pinot Noir)
- ❖ 2 cups beef broth
- ❖ 1 tablespoon Worcestershire sauce
- ❖ 2 bay leaves
- ❖ 1 teaspoon dried thyme
- ❖ 2 tablespoons flour
- ❖ 2 tablespoons butter, softened
- ❖ Fresh parsley, chopped (for garnish)

INSTRUCTIONS

Cook the Bacon:

1. Cook cubed bacon in a large skillet over medium heat until crispy. Transfer the bacon to the slow cooker while still in the skillet.
2. Best to
3. Brown Beef: Season beef cubes with salt and pepper. Cook the meat in batches over medium-high heat in the same

skillet until browned. Browned beef goes in the slow cooker.

4. Add the pearl onions, garlic, carrots, celery, and mushrooms to the same skillet and sauté the vegetables. When the vegetables begin to soften, sauté them for about five minutes. After adding the tomato paste, simmer for an additional minute. After that, move the veggies to the slow cooker.
5. Pour the red wine into the skillet and bring it to a simmer, scraping off any browned bits from the pan's bottom. This will deglaze the skillet. Pour the wine into the slow cooker.
6. Include the Remaining Ingredients: Fill the slow cooker with the Worcestershire sauce, bay leaves, thyme, and beef broth. Mix well to blend.

Cook:

1. After cooking the meat, cover and simmer for 8–10 hours on low or 4–6 hours on high.
2. Pour the Sauce Down: About 30 minutes before serving, make a smooth paste (beurre manié) by combining flour and softened butter. This mixture, when added to the slow cooker, will cause the sauce to coagulate. Return the heat to high and proceed with the cooking process.

Completing and serving:

1. Take out the bay leaves from the cooker on low heat.
2. After tasting it, add more salt and pepper to the stew's flavoring.
3. Garnish the Beef Bourguignon with freshly cut parsley and serve it hot. Mashed potatoes, egg noodles, or crusty toast go nicely with it.

- ➤ Wine Selection: Go with a good red wine for the most flavor. Although dry red wine can do the trick, Burgundy or Pinot Noir are classic options.
- ➤ Other Root veggies: If preferred, you can use turnips or parsnips for the different root veggies.
- ➤ Pearl Onions: To facilitate peeling, blanch fresh pearl onions for one minute in boiling water before putting them in an ice bath.
- ➤ Storage: Beef Bourguignon leftovers can be frozen for up to three months or refrigerated for up to three days in an airtight container. Before serving, could you give them a thorough heat?
- ➤ Beurre Manié: The Sauce can be thickened without forming lumps by combining flour and butter. Before adding to the slow cooker, ensure the mixture is smooth and the butter has softened.
- ➤ Enjoy your classic and flavorful slow-cooked Beef Bourguignon!

34 | P a g e

9. SLOW COOKER JAMBALAYA

INGREDIENTS:

- ❖ Cover and boil until the chicken is done and the rice is soft, 2–3 hours on High or 4–6 hours on Low.
- ❖ 1 pound smoked sausage, sliced
- ❖ 1 pound shrimp, peeled and deveined
- ❖ 1 onion, chopped
- ❖ 1 green bell pepper, chopped
- ❖ 2 stalks celery, chopped
- ❖ 3 cloves garlic, minced
- ❖ 1 can (14.5 ounces) diced tomatoes, undrained
- ❖ 1 can (6 ounces) tomato paste
- ❖ 3 cups chicken broth
- ❖ 1 cup long-grain white rice
- ❖ 2 teaspoons Cajun seasoning
- ❖ 1 teaspoon dried thyme
- ❖ 1 teaspoon dried oregano
- ❖ 1 teaspoon paprika
- ❖ 1/2 teaspoon cayenne pepper (adjust to taste)
- ❖ Salt and pepper to taste
- ❖ Chopped fresh parsley (for garnish)
- ❖ Sliced green onions (for garnish)

INSTRUCTIONS:

1. Prepare the ingredients by chopping the garlic, onion, bell pepper, and celery.
2. Cut the smoked sausage into round pieces.
3. Roughly chop the chicken thighs into small pieces.
4. If you haven't already, peel and devein the shrimp.

5. Add all ingredients to the slow cooker.
6. Add the shrimp, diced onion, bell pepper, celery, minced garlic, and smoked sausage to the slow cooker and the chicken thighs.
7. Add the rice, thyme, oregano, paprika, cayenne pepper, tomato paste, diced tomatoes, chicken stock, and Cajun seasoning. Mix thoroughly to blend.

Cook:

- ➢ Cover and boil until the chicken is done and the rice is soft, 2–3 hours on High or 4–6 hours on Low.
- ➢ Taste after cooking and season as needed.
- ➢ Add chopped green onions and fresh parsley and serve hot.

NOTES:

Variations:

- ➢ Add chopped ham, diced tomatoes with green chilies, or okra to make your jambalaya unique.

Spice Level:

- ➢ Modify the cayenne pepper quantity to suit your heat tolerance.

Rice:

- ➢ For optimal effects, use long-grain white rice. You can also use brown rice; however, you might need to change the amount of liquid and boiling time.

Seafood:

➤ You can use a mixture of crawfish tails, crab meat, and shrimp for the seafood component.

Storage:

➤ You may freeze leftover jambalaya for up to three months or keep it in the refrigerator for up to three days when kept in an airtight container. Thoroughly reheat before serving.
➤ Savor your flavorful and filling jambalaya, simmered!

10. SLOW COOKER COQ AU VIN

INGREDIENTS:

- ❖ Six slices bacon, chopped
- ❖ 4 chicken thighs, bone-in, skin-on
- ❖ 4 chicken drumsticks, bone-in, skin-on
- ❖ Salt and pepper to taste
- ❖ 1 onion, chopped
- ❖ 2 cloves garlic, minced
- ❖ 8 ounces mushrooms, sliced
- ❖ 1 cup carrots, chopped
- ❖ 1 cup chicken broth
- ❖ 2 cups Burgundy or Pinot Noir
- ❖ 2 tablespoons tomato paste
- ❖ 2 bay leaves
- ❖ 1 teaspoon dried thyme
- ❖ 1 teaspoon dried rosemary
- ❖ 1 tablespoon all-purpose flour
- ❖ 2 tablespoons butter
- ❖ Chopped fresh parsley for garnish

INSTRUCTIONS:

Cook

1. diced bacon in a pan over medium heat until crispy. Leave bacon fat in the skillet as you carefully remove

it with a slotted spoon.

1. Salt and pepper drumsticks and thighs to brown. All sides of bacon grease skillet chicken should be golden brown. Put chicken in a low-heat cooker.

To sauté vegetables

1. , add chopped onion, minced garlic, mushrooms, and diced carrots to the same skillet. After a few minutes of sautéing, the vegetables should soften. Cook veggies in slow cooker.
2. Add liquid and seasonings.
3. Put red wine and chicken stock in the slow cooker.
4. Stir in dried thyme, rosemary, bay leaves, and tomato paste.
5. Simmer: Cover and s
6. immer the chicken for 6–8 hours on Low or 3–4 hours on High until tender.
7. Make a smooth paste (beurre manié) of flour and butter 30 minutes before cooking to thicken the sauce. Stir this paste into the slow cooker and keep cooking until the sauce thickens.
8. After cooking, taste the sauce and add salt and pepper to suit.
9. Serve the Coq au Vin hot, topped with chopped fresh parsley and crispy bacon. It goes nicely with noodles, crusty bread, or mashed potatoes.

- Choose a high-quality red wine like Pinot Noir or Burgundy for authentic flavor.
- Variations with Vegetables: Feel free to include different veggies, including potatoes or pearl onions.
- Chicken: Cooking the meal with bone-in, skin-on chicken chunks enhances taste and moisture.
- Storage: Leftover coq au vin may be frozen for up to three months or kept in the refrigerator for up to three days in an airtight container. Thoroughly reheat before serving.

INGREDIENTS:

- ❖ 3-4 pounds pork shoulder (also known as pork butt), trimmed of excess fat
- ❖ 1 large onion, thinly sliced
- ❖ 4 cloves garlic, minced
- ❖ 1 cup barbecue sauce (plus extra for serving)
- ❖ 1/2 cup chicken broth or water
- ❖ 2 tablespoons brown sugar
- ❖ 2 tablespoons apple cider vinegar
- ❖ 1 tablespoon Worcestershire sauce
- ❖ 1 tablespoon mustard (optional)
- ❖ 1 teaspoon smoked paprika
- ❖ 1 teaspoon chili powder
- ❖ Salt and pepper, to taste
- ❖ Hamburger buns or rolls for serving

INSTRUCTIONS:

Get the pork ready:

> ➤ Liberally season it with salt and pepper after removing extra fat from the pork shoulder.

In the Slow Cooker, layer:

1. Put the minced garlic and sliced onion in the slow cooker's bottom.
2. Place the spiced pork shoulder over the garlic and onions.

3. In a bowl, stir brown sugar, apple cider vinegar, Worcestershire sauce, smoked paprika, chili powder, and chicken broth (or water).
4. Pour Sauce on Pork: Evenly cover pork shoulder with barbecue sauce.

After

1. the pork is tender and easily shredded with a fork, cook on low for 8-10 hours or high for 4-6 hours.
2. Remove the pork shoulder and place it on a chopping board to shred.
3. Use two forks to shred pork into bite-sized chunks. Remove excess fat.
4. Simmer the slow cooker liquid in a pan over medium heat to thicken the sauce. The thickened sauce can be added to pulled pork.
5. Add sauce: Return the shredded pork to the slow cooker and add the thickened sauce.

Serve:

➢ Spoon the pulled pork with barbecue sauce over hamburger buns or rolls if preferred.

NOTES:

➢ Pork Shoulder: Slow-cooking pork shoulder renders it moist and soft, making it the perfect cut for pulled pork.
➢ Barbecue Sauce: Use your preferred homemade or store-bought sauce for extra taste.
➢ Personalization: You can adjust the sauce and seasoning to your tastes. You can increase the amount of spices, change the sweetness, or increase the heat.

➤ Storage: Any leftover pulled pork can be frozen for up to three months or kept in the refrigerator for up to three days when kept in an airtight container. Before serving, reheat.

INGREDIENTS:

- ❖ 4-6 bone-in, skin-on chicken thighs or drumsticks
- ❖ Salt and pepper, to taste
- ❖ 2 tablespoons olive oil
- ❖ 1 onion, thinly sliced
- ❖ 3 cloves garlic, minced
- ❖ 1 bell pepper, sliced (any color)
- ❖ 1 cup sliced mushrooms
- ❖ 1 can (14.5 ounces) diced tomatoes, undrained
- ❖ 1 can (6 ounces) tomato paste
- ❖ 1/2 cup chicken broth or dry red wine
- ❖ 1 teaspoon dried oregano
- ❖ 1 teaspoon dried basil
- ❖ 1/2 teaspoon dried thyme
- ❖ 1/2 teaspoon dried rosemary
- ❖ 1 bay leaf
- ❖ 1/4 cup of freshly chopped parsley for garnish
- ❖ Cooked pasta or crusty bread for serving

INSTRUCTIONS:

Season

1. chicken drumsticks and thighs with salt and pepper.
1. Sear chicken in olive oil in a large skillet over medium-high heat. It should be browned for 3-4 minutes per side. After browning, cook the chicken in the slow cooker.

Vegetable

1. Sauté: Add bell pepper, onion, mushrooms, and minced garlic to the same skillet. Sauté until tender, about 5 minutes.

Add everything to the slow cooker.

1. Add browned chicken and sautéed vegetables to the slow cooker.
2. Add chopped tomatoes, tomato paste, wine or chicken broth, dried oregano, rosemary, thyme, and bay leaf in the slow cooker. Mix all ingredients.

Cook:

1. Cover and simmer the chicken for 6–8 hours on Low or 3–4 hours on High until soft and done.
1. Remove the slow cooker
2. bay leaf and serve after cooking.
3. Add salt and pepper to taste.
4. Add fresh parsley to Chicken Cacciatore. Serve sauce over spaghetti or crusty bread to soak up.

NOTES:

> Chicken: This recipe can use bone-in, skin-on chicken thighs or drumsticks. Chicken breasts can also be used, but they may cook faster and become dry, so adjust the cooking time accordingly.
> Vegetables: Feel free to add other vegetables, such as olives, zucchini, or carrots.

- ➢ Wine Substitute: If you choose not to use wine, add water or chicken broth.
- ➢ Storage: Leftover chicken cacciatore may be frozen for up to three months or kept in the refrigerator for up to three days when kept in an airtight container. Thoroughly reheat before serving.

INGREDIENTS:

- ❖ Each measuring approximately 1 1/2 inches thick, four veal shanks were fastened around the bone using kitchen thread.
- ❖ Salt and pepper to taste
- ❖ 1/2 cup all-purpose flour for dredging
- ❖ 2 tablespoons olive oil
- ❖ 1 onion, finely chopped
- ❖ 2 carrots, finely chopped
- ❖ 2 celery stalks, finely chopped
- ❖ 4 cloves garlic, minced
- ❖ 1 cup dry white wine
- ❖ 1 can (14.5 ounces) diced tomatoes, undrained
- ❖ 1 cup beef or veal broth
- ❖ 2 bay leaves
- ❖ 1 teaspoon dried thyme
- ❖ 1 teaspoon dried rosemary
- ❖ 1/2 teaspoon dried oregano
- ❖ Gremolata (optional for serving):
- ❖ Zest of 1 lemon
- ❖ 2 tablespoons chopped fresh parsley
- ❖ 1 clove garlic, minced

INSTRUCTIONS:

1. To prepare the veal shanks, season them liberally with salt and pepper. After coating them with flour, shake off any extra flour.
2. Melt the olive oil in a big skillet over medium-high heat for vegetable shank roasting. Take around 3 to 4 minutes to brown each side of the veal shanks. Shanks should be transferred to the slow cooker after browning.
3. Chop the onion, carrots, celery, and minced garlic and add them to the same skillet for sautéing vegetables. Cook for approximately five minutes or until the veggies are tender.
4. Remove burnt parts from the pan's bottom by adding the white wine to the skillet and scraping it around. The wine will diminish slightly if it simmers for a few minutes.
5. Add ingredients to slow cooker and stir.
6. Add the browned veal shanks to the slow cooker, the veggies that have been sautéed, and the wine deglazed.
7. In the slow cooker, toss the chopped tomatoes (with their juices), dried thyme, dried rosemary, dried oregano, bay leaves, and beef or veal broth to mix.
8. Simmer the veal for 6–8 hours on Low or 3–4 hours on High until tender and easily pulled from the bone. Cover when cooking.
9. Produce Gremolata (Optional):
10. Gently stir the minced garlic, fresh parsley, and lemon zest in a small bowl. The classic topping for Osso Buco is this gremolata.
11. Discard the bay leaves and remove the cooked veal shanks from the slow cooker before serving. Serving suggestions: If preferred, serve hot Osso Buco with mashed potatoes, polenta, or risotto and gremolata.

NOTES:

➢ Veal Shank Substitution: If veal isn't available, shanks made from beef or lamb can be substituted; however, the flavor will alter slightly.

➢ Option 2: Increase the quantity of beef or veal broth and eliminate the wine if you would instead not use any.

➢ Storage: Leftover Osso Buco can be refrigerated or frozen for three days or up to three months when kept in an airtight container. Stir it well before serving.

INGREDIENTS:

- ❖ 1 large butternut squash (about 3 pounds), peeled, seeded, and cubed
- ❖ 1 onion, chopped
- ❖ 2 carrots, chopped
- ❖ 2 celery stalks, chopped
- ❖ 3 cloves garlic, minced
- ❖ 4 cups vegetable broth
- ❖ 1 teaspoon ground cumin
- ❖ 1/2 teaspoon ground cinnamon
- ❖ 1/4 teaspoon ground nutmeg
- ❖ Salt and pepper to taste
- ❖ 1/2 cup coconut milk or substantial cream (optional)
- ❖ Fresh parsley or chives, chopped (for garnish)
- ❖ Toasted pumpkin seeds (pepitas) for garnish (optional)

INSTRUCTIONS:

Get the ingredients ready:

1. Butternut squash should be peeled, seeded, and cubed.
2. Chop the garlic, celery, carrots, and onion.
3. Add all ingredients to the slow cooker.
4. Add the diced onion, celery, carrots, cubed butternut squash, and minced garlic to the slow cooker.
5. Add the broth made of vegetables.
6. Incorporate the ground nutmeg, cinnamon, and cumin.
7. Season with salt and pepper to taste.

Simmer:

1. Cover and simmer until the vegetables are extremely soft, 6 to 8 hours on Low or 3 to 4 hours on High.

Blend Soup:

1. After the veggies are cooked, blend the soup until it's smooth using an immersion blender. Alternatively, gently transfer the soup to a blender, puree it until it's soft, and then put it back into the slow cooker.

Cream (Optional):

1. Stir heavy cream or coconut milk into pureed soup until thoroughly blended. This will give the soup more creaminess and richness.
2. Salt and pepper the soup to taste.
3. Divide butternut squash soup into bowls.
4. Add roasted pumpkin seeds and finely chopped fresh parsley or chives if desired.
5. If desired, serve hot with croutons or crusty toast.

NOTES:

➢ Add thyme, curry powder, or ginger to customize the soup.
➢ Coconut milk can replace heavy cream for a rich mouthfeel without dairy.
➢ Storage: Leftover butternut squash soup can be frozen for up to three months or kept in the refrigerator for up to four days in an airtight container. Before serving, reheat.

15. COOKER BAKED BEANS

INGREDIENTS:

- ❖ 1-pound dried navy beans, washed and soaked overnight
- ❖ 1 onion, finely chopped
- ❖ 4 cloves garlic, minced
- ❖ 1/2 cup ketchup
- ❖ 1/2 cup molasses
- ❖ 1/4 cup brown sugar
- ❖ 2 tablespoons yellow mustard
- ❖ 1 tablespoon Worcestershire sauce
- ❖ 1 teaspoon smoked paprika
- ❖ 1 teaspoon salt
- ❖ 1/2 teaspoon black pepper
- ❖ 4 cups water or vegetable broth
- ❖ 4 slices bacon, chopped (optional for added flavor)

INSTRUCTIONS:

1. Soak the Beans: Fill a big dish with rinsed dried navy beans. Cover the beans with water and soak them for the entire night. Drain and rinse the beans before using.
2. Mince garlic and cut onion.
3. In a slow cooker, combine soaked navy beans, smoked paprika, chopped onion, minced garlic, ketchup, molasses, brown sugar, yellow mustard, Worcestershire sauce, salt, and black pepper.
4. Add the chopped bacon to the slow cooker if you're using it.
5. Add Liquid: Make sure the beans are entirely immersed by adding the water or vegetable broth.

6. Cook: Cover and cook low for 8–10 hours or high for 4–6 hours until beans are cooked and sauce thick.
7. If necessary, taste the baked beans and adjust the spice. Add more salt, pepper, or other herbs to taste.
8. Serve: Warm baked beans can be served as an accompaniment to sandwiches, grilled meats, or any barbecue spread.

NOTES:

➢ Bacon Substitute: If you're a vegetarian baked bean lover, you can substitute bacon with veggie broth in place of water to increase flavor.
➢ Add extra items to the baked beans, like chopped bell peppers, jalapeños, or even a little apple cider vinegar for some tang.
➢ Storage: The remaining baked beans can be kept in the fridge in an airtight container for up to four days—reheat before serving.

16. SLOW COOKER MINESTRONE SOUP

INGREDIENTS:

- ❖ 1 onion, chopped
- ❖ 2 carrots, diced
- ❖ 2 celery stalks, diced
- ❖ 3 cloves garlic, minced
- ❖ 1 can (14.5 ounces) diced tomatoes, undrained
- ❖ 1 can (15 ounces) kidney beans, drained and rinsed
- ❖ 1-can (15-ounce) drained and washed cannellini beans
- ❖ 4 cups vegetable broth
- ❖ 2 cups water
- ❖ 1 teaspoon dried basil
- ❖ 1 teaspoon dried oregano
- ❖ 1/2 teaspoon dried thyme
- ❖ 1 bay leaf
- ❖ Salt and pepper to taste
- ❖ 1 cup ditalini or tiny shell pasta
- ❖ 2 cups chopped fresh spinach or kale
- ❖ Grated Parmesan cheese for serving (optional)
- ❖ Crusty bread for serving

INSTRUCTIONS:

1. Chop the onion, dice the carrots, dice the celery, mince the garlic, dice the tomatoes, kidney beans, cannellini beans, vegetable broth, water, dried basil, dried oregano, dried thyme, bay leaf, salt, and pepper in the slow cooker.
2. Cook: Cover and cook for 6–8 hours on Low or 3–4 hours on High, or until the veggies are soft and the flavors are well combined.

3. Add the pasta and greens: Stir in the small pasta about 30 minutes before the soup is finished cooking. Pasta should be cooked until al dente.
4. Add the finely chopped kale or spinach and simmer until it wilts.
5. Adjust seasoning by tasting the soup and adding salt and pepper.
6. Divide the soup into bowls to serve.
7. If preferred, top hot servings with grated Parmesan cheese.
8. Savor with some crusty bread for a filling dinner.

NOTES:

➤ Variations: Because minestrone may be made with many different veggies, you can add green beans, potatoes, or zucchini.
➤ Beans: Feel free to use whatever variety of beans you enjoy or have on hand, such as black beans, navy beans, or chickpeas.
➤ Pasta: To avoid mushy pasta, add the pasta after cooking.
➤ Storage: Refrigerate leftover minestrone for four days and reheat before serving.

INGREDIENTS:

- ❖ Rinsed and sorted 1 pound (2 cups) dry split peas
- ❖ 1 onion, chopped
- ❖ 2 carrots, diced
- ❖ 2 celery stalks, diced
- ❖ 3 cloves garlic, minced
- ❖ 8 cups vegetable or chicken broth
- ❖ 1 bay leaf
- ❖ 1 teaspoon dried thyme
- ❖ 1/2 teaspoon dried rosemary
- ❖ Salt and pepper, to taste
- ❖ Optional toppings: crispy bacon, chopped ham, chopped parsley, sour cream

INSTRUCTIONS:

1. Add all ingredients to the slow cooker.
2. In the slow cooker, add the rinsed and sorted dried split peas, chopped onion, diced carrots, celery, minced garlic, bay leaf, dried thyme, and dried rosemary.
3. Add the chicken or veggie broth.
4. Simmer: Cover and cook split peas for 8–10 hours on Low or 4–6 hours on High
5. until tender.
6. Use an immersion blender after cooking the split peas for a smooth soup. Or, you can.
7. Adjust seasoning by tasting the soup and adding salt and pepper.
8. Pour the split pea soup into individual dishes.

9. Optional garnishes include diced ham, crispy bacon, chopped parsley, or a dollop of sour cream.
10. Serve hot with crackers or crusty bread on the side.

NOTES:

➢ Variations: For more taste and texture, add other ingredients like diced potatoes, minced ham hock, or smoked sausage.
➢ Thickness: Use a potato masher to mash some split peas to thicken the soup.
➢ Storage: Leftover split pea soup can be kept in the fridge for up to four days by placing it in an airtight container— reheat before serving.

18. SLOW COOKER RED BEANS AND RICE

INGREDIENTS:

- ❖ 1 pound dried red kidney beans and rinsed and sorted
- ❖ 1 onion, chopped
- ❖ 2 celery stalks, chopped
- ❖ 1 green bell pepper, chopped
- ❖ 3 cloves garlic, minced
- ❖ 1 pound smoked sausage, sliced (such as Andouille)
- ❖ 4 cups chicken broth
- ❖ 2 cups water
- ❖ 1 tablespoon Cajun seasoning
- ❖ 1 teaspoon dried thyme
- ❖ 1 teaspoon dried oregano
- ❖ 1/2 teaspoon smoked paprika
- ❖ 1/4 teaspoon cayenne pepper (adjust to taste)
- ❖ Salt and pepper, to taste
- ❖ Cooked white rice for serving
- ❖ Chopped green onions for garnish

INSTRUCTIONS:

1. You can soak dry red kidney beans overnight or use the fast soak method, which involves boiling the water and beans for an hour before draining them.
2. Put ingredients in slow cooker:
3. Simmer red kidney beans (drain if not soaked) with water, chicken stock, Cajun spice, dry paprika, dried thyme, and cayenne pepper. Add chopped celery, onion, green bell pepper, minced garlic, and smoked sausage.

4. Simmer: Cover and simmer for 8–10 hours on Low or 4–6 hours on High until the beans are soft and creamy.

5. Optional: Mash some beans against the slow cooker side with a potato masher to thicken.

6. Taste the red beans and rice and add salt, pepper, cayenne, or Cajun flavor if needed.

7. Serving suggestions: hot red beans and rice over cooked white rice.

8. Garnish with chopped green onions before serving.

NOTE:

➢ While any smoked sausage can be used, andouille sausage is typically used with red beans and rice.

➢ To make Cajun spice, mix paprika, cayenne, onion, garlic, and thyme with black pepper, or buy it.

➢ Variations: Add bell peppers, diced tomatoes, or sliced ham for flavor and texture.

➢ Red beans and rice can be refrigerated for 4 days in an airtight jar. Reheat before serving.

INGREDIENTS:

- 1 pounds of skinless, boneless chicken breasts sliced into small pieces
- 1 onion, finely chopped
- 4 cloves garlic, minced
- 1 tablespoon fresh ginger, grated
- 1 can (14.5 oz) diced tomatoes
- 1 can (14 oz) coconut milk
- 1/4 cup tomato paste
- 2 tablespoons ghee or vegetable oil
- 2 tablespoons garam masala
- 1 tablespoon ground coriander
- 1 tablespoon ground cumin
- 1 teaspoon ground turmeric
- 1 teaspoon paprika
- 1 teaspoon ground cinnamon
- 1/2 teaspoon cayenne pepper (adjust to taste)
- Salt and pepper to taste
- 1/4 cup plain Greek yogurt
- Fresh cilantro, chopped (for garnish)
- Cooked rice or naan for serving

INSTRUCTIONS:

1. To sauté aromatics, place a skillet over medium heat with either ghee or vegetable oil. Simmer the chopped onion for approximately five minutes or until it becomes tender. Add the minced garlic and grated ginger and cook for another minute or two or until fragrant.
2. Add all ingredients to the slow cooker.
3. Add the ginger, garlic, and onion that have been sautéed to the slow cooker. Diced tomatoes, coconut milk, tomato paste, paprika, ground cinnamon, cayenne pepper, ground coriander, ground cumin, ground turmeric, and salt and pepper should all be added. Mix everything.
4. Add Chicken: Transfer the trim pieces to the slow cooker and stir to distribute the sauce evenly.
5. Cook: Cover and simmer on Low for 6–8 hours or High for 3–4 hours until chicken is soft and cooked.
6. Thicken Sauce: To thicken the sauce, stir in the plain Greek yogurt about 30 minutes before the cooking time is over. Stir thoroughly until adequately combined.

Serve:

➢ Warm chicken tikka masala with nan bread or over-boiled rice.
➢ Before serving, add some freshly cut cilantro as a garnish.

NOTES:

- ➢ For extra taste and tenderness, use skinless, boneless chicken thighs instead of breasts.
- ➢ Spice Level: To suit your taste, reduce or increase the cayenne pepper in the recipe.
- ➢ Storage: Leftover chicken tikka masala can be frozen for up to three months or kept in the refrigerator for up to three days in an airtight container—reheat before serving.

INGREDIENTS:

- ❖ Four large bell peppers (any color), cut off the tops and seeds
- ❖ Lean ground beef pound
- ❖ 1 cup cooked rice (white or brown)
- ❖ 1 onion, finely chopped
- ❖ 2 cloves garlic, minced
- ❖ 1 can (14.5 ounces) diced tomatoes, drained
- ❖ 1 cup tomato sauce
- ❖ 1 teaspoon dried oregano
- ❖ 1 teaspoon dried basil
- ❖ 1/2 teaspoon paprika
- ❖ Salt and pepper to taste
- ❖ One cup of finely shredded mozzarella cheese
- ❖ Freshly chopped basil or parsley (optional)

INSTRUCTIONS:

1. To remove the seeds and membranes, cut off the tops of the bell peppers. Give the peppers a brief rinse under cold water and leave aside.
2. To brown the filling, thoroughly sear the ground beef in a skillet over medium heat. Trim off any extra fat as needed.
3. Add the minced garlic and onion pieces to the same skillet. Cook for 3–4 minutes, or until tender.
4. Incorporate cooked rice, chopped tomatoes, tomato sauce, paprika, dried basil and oregano, and adjust the seasoning with salt and pepper. Add the remaining 2 to 3 minutes of simmering time to help the flavors come together.

5. Ladle the ingredients evenly into each hollowed-out pepper and gently press down to firmly press the bell pepper contents inside.
6. Utilize the Slow Cooker: Place the bell peppers in the slow cooker vertically to ensure they are strong and won't collapse while cooking.
7. stew: Cook, covered, until the bell peppers are very soft, 6 to 8 hours on Low or 3 to 4 hours on High.
8. Add Cheese: Top the stuffed bell peppers with shredded mozzarella cheese fifteen to twenty minutes before the cooking procedure is complete. Cover and warm the cheese until it bubbles and melts.

Serve:

➤ Take the filled bell peppers out of the slow cooker and transfer them to serving platters with care.
➤ If desired, garnish with finely chopped fresh basil or parsley.
➤ Enjoy while hot!

NOTES:

➤ Variations: You can change the dish by adding quinoa, corn, black beans, or diced tomatoes.
➤ Vegetarian Option: Cooked lentils or quinoa can be used in place of ground beef to create a vegetarian version of stuffed bell peppers.
➤ Storage: Store any leftover stuffed bell peppers in the refrigerator in an airtight container for up to three days. Reheat before serving.

INGREDIENTS:

- ❖ 1 lb (450g) boneless, skinless chicken breasts
- ❖ One 14.5-oz can of chopped tomatoes
- ❖ One can (14.5 oz) of rinsed and drained black beans
- ❖ 1 can (14.5 oz) corn kernels, drained
- ❖ 1 onion, chopped
- ❖ 1 red bell pepper, chopped
- ❖ 1 green bell pepper, chopped
- ❖ 2 cloves garlic, minced
- ❖ 4 cups (946ml) chicken broth
- ❖ 1 teaspoon chili powder
- ❖ 1 teaspoon cumin
- ❖ 1 teaspoon paprika
- ❖ Salt and pepper to taste
- ❖ Juice of 1 lime
- ❖ 1/4 cup chopped fresh cilantro
- ❖ Tortilla chips, shredded cheese, avocado slices, and sour cream for serving (optional)

INSTRUCTIONS:

1. Place chicken breasts in slow cooker bottom.
2. Put diced tomatoes, juices, black beans, corn, onion, bell peppers, and garlic in the slow cooker.
3. Cover slow cooker ingredients with chicken stock.
4. Season the slow cooker
5. with chili powder, cumin, paprika, salt, and pepper.
6. When the chicken is tender, cover it and simmer for 6–8 hours on low or 3–4 hours on high.

7. After taking the chicken breasts out of the slow cooker, shred them with two forks. Refill the slow cooker with shredded chicken.
8. Stir in chopped cilantro and lime juice. Taste and season as needed.
9. Cheese shreds, tortilla chips, sour cream, and avocado slices can be added to the steaming casserole.

NOTE:

➢ You can change this recipe by adding cooked rice, chopped green chiles, or jalapenos.
➢ If you want a thicker soup, you can purée a portion with an immersion blender before adding the shredded chicken.
➢ The remaining food can be refrigerated in an airtight container for up to three days.

22. PORK RIBS

INGREDIENTS:

- ❖ Two racks of pork ribs weighing a combined 4–5 pounds
- ❖ 1 cup barbecue sauce (store-bought or homemade)
- ❖ 1/4 cup apple cider vinegar
- ❖ 1/4 cup brown sugar
- ❖ 2 cloves garlic, minced
- ❖ 1 teaspoon smoked paprika
- ❖ 1 teaspoon onion powder
- ❖ 1 teaspoon garlic powder
- ❖ Salt and pepper to taste
- ❖ Green onions or fresh parsley, chopped (optional)

INSTRUCTIONS:

1. If desired, remove the thin membrane from the back of the ribs for better flavor penetration. Season the ribs liberally with salt, pepper, smoked paprika, onion powder, and garlic powder.
2. Combine the brown sugar, apple cider vinegar, minced garlic, and barbecue sauce in a bowl.
3. Place the ribs in the slow cooker, on the meaty side, on the outside and pile them against the walls.
4. Make sure the ribs are evenly coated with the barbecue sauce as you pour it over them.
5. Cover and stew the ribs for 6–8 hours on low or 3–4 hours on high, or until they are soft and cooked through.
6. When the ribs are done, carefully take them out of the slow cooker and put them on a foil-covered baking sheet.
7. Set the oven's broiler on high.

8. Brush the ribs with some of the sauce from the slow cooker and broil until the sauce is bubbling and caramelized about three to five minutes.
9. Remove the ribs from the oven and give them a few minutes to rest before slicing them into individual plates.
10. If preferred, top with finely chopped green onions or fresh parsley and serve hot.

NOTE:

➢ You can alter the taste of the ribs by varying the barbecue sauce brand or adding extra seasonings to the sauce blend.
➢ For extra flavor, sprinkle the ribs with your favorite dry rub before placing them in the slow cooker.
➢ For up to three days, leftover ribs should be in an airtight container in the refrigerator.

23. BEEF BRISKET

INGREDIENTS:

- ❖ 3-4 pounds (1.4-1.8 kg) beef brisket
- ❖ 2 onions, sliced
- ❖ 4 cloves garlic, minced
- ❖ 1 cup beef broth
- ❖ 1/2 cup barbecue sauce
- ❖ 1/4 cup soy sauce
- ❖ 2 tablespoons Worcestershire sauce
- ❖ 2 tablespoons brown sugar
- ❖ 2 teaspoons smoked paprika
- ❖ 1 teaspoon ground mustard
- ❖ 1 teaspoon dried thyme
- ❖ To taste, add salt and pepper.
- ❖ Garnish with optional chopped green onions or fresh parsley.

INSTRUCTIONS:

1. Use a lot of salt, pepper, smoked paprika, and ground mustard to season the beef brisket.
2. Combine the soy sauce, Worcestershire sauce, brown sugar, dried thyme, barbecue sauce, and beef broth in a bowl.
3. Put the minced garlic and sliced onions in the slow cooker's bottom.
4. Top the onions and garlic with the spiced beef brisket.
5. Please ensure the brisket is evenly coated after pouring the sauce mixture over it.

6. When the brisket is fork-tender, cook it covered for 8–10 hours on low or 4–6 hours on high.
7. After cooking, carefully take the brisket from the slow cooker and place it on a chopping board. Wait a few minutes before slicing against the grain.
8. Spoon some of the sauce over the top, and serve the sliced brisket with the onions and garlic from the slow cooker.
9. If preferred, garnish with finely chopped green onions or fresh parsley and serve hot.

NOTE:

➤ You can alter the brisket's flavor by incorporating extra seasonings into the sauce mixture or using your preferred barbecue sauce.
➤ Before putting the brisket in the slow cooker, sear it in a hot skillet for more flavor.
➤ Brisket leftovers can be frozen for three months or refrigerated for three days in an airtight container.

INGREDIENTS:

- ❖ 1 large eggplant, diced
- ❖ 2 medium zucchinis, diced
- ❖ 1 large onion, diced
- ❖ 2 bell peppers (red, yellow, or green), diced
- ❖ 3 cloves garlic, minced
- ❖ 4 large tomatoes, diced
- ❖ 2 tablespoons tomato paste
- ❖ 2 teaspoons dried thyme
- ❖ 2 teaspoons dried basil
- ❖ Salt and pepper to taste
- ❖ Olive oil
- ❖ Fresh basil leaves, torn (for garnish, optional)

INSTRUCTIONS:

1. Get 1 tablespoon of olive oil hot in a skillet over medium heat. Brown the eggplant by frying it for 5 minutes. Slow simmer the eggplant.
2. If necessary, add chopped onion, zucchini, bell peppers, and extra tablespoon of olive oil to the skillet. In order to achieve tenderness, cook for approximately seven to seven minutes. Stir the
3. ingredients and place in the slow cooker.
4. Add diced tomatoes, dried basil, dry thyme, and minced garlic to the slow cooker. Mix ingredients well.
5. Season with salt and pepper to taste.
6. After the vegetables are tender but not mushy, cover and cook on low for 6–8 hours or high for 3–4 hours.

7. Taste and seasonbefore serving.
8. Add freshly torn basil leaves before serving.

NOTE:

> ➢ Can be Ratatouille Used as a side, topping crusty bread, or with pasta, rice, or quinoa. It tastes nice cold at normal temperature.
> ➢ You can add carrots or mushrooms to taste.
> ➢ Refrigerate leftovers for three to four days. Ratatouille makes a good freezer food. Reheat gently in the microwave or stove before serving.

25. SAUSAGE AND SAUERKRAUT

INGREDIENTS:

- ❖ 1 package (about 1 pound) of your favorite sausages (such as bratwurst, kielbasa, or smoked sausage)
- ❖ 1 pound sauerkraut, drained and rinsed
- ❖ 1 onion, thinly sliced
- ❖ 2 cloves garlic, minced
- ❖ 1 teaspoon caraway seeds (optional)
- ❖ 1 cup chicken broth or beer
- ❖ Salt and pepper to taste
- ❖ Mustard for serving (optional)
- ❖ Chopped fresh parsley for garnish (optional)

INSTRUCTIONS:

1. Brown raw sausages in a skillet over medium heat for a few minutes on each side to enhance flavor. You can skip this step.
2. Sausages, sauerkraut, diced onion, minced garlic, and caraway seeds
3. go in the slow cooker.
4. Pour chicken broth or beer over the slow cooker contents.
5. Season with salt and pepper to taste.
6. Sausage should be tender after 6–8 hours of low cooking or 3–4 hours of vigorous cooking. Cover and cook.
7. Taste and season before serving.
8. Hot sausages with sauerkraut can be served alone or with mustard for dipping. Add fresh parsley if desired.

NOTE:

> ➤ This dish can be customized by adding sliced potatoes or apples for flavor and texture.
> ➤ Refrigerate leftovers for three to four days. Reheat gently in the microwave or stove before serving.

INGREDIENTS:

- ❖ 4 bone-in, skinless chicken thighs (or any chicken pieces you prefer)
- ❖ 1 onion, finely chopped
- ❖ 3 cloves garlic, minced
- ❖ 1 teaspoon ground cumin
- ❖ 1 teaspoon ground coriander
- ❖ 1 teaspoon paprika
- ❖ 1/2 teaspoon ground cinnamon
- ❖ 1/2 teaspoon ground ginger
- ❖ 1/4 teaspoon ground turmeric
- ❖ Pinch of cayenne pepper (adjust to taste)
- ❖ 1 can (14 ounces) diced tomatoes, undrained
- ❖ 1 cup chicken broth
- ❖ 1/2 cup dried apricots, chopped
- ❖ 1/4 cup raisins
- ❖ 2 tablespoons tomato paste
- ❖ Salt and pepper to taste
- ❖ Fresh cilantro, chopped (for garnish)
- ❖ Cooked couscous or rice for serving

INSTRUCTIONS:

1. Mix ground cumin, coriander, ginger, turmeric, cinnamon, paprika, and cayenne pepper in a bowl.
2. Rub the spice mixture evenly on the chicken thighs.
3. Cook chicken thighs in the slow cooker.
4. Diced dried apricots, raisins, tomatoes, onion, garlic, and tomato paste go in the slow cooker.

5. Season with salt and pepper to taste.
6. When the chicken is tender, For 6–8 hours on low or 3–4 hours on high, cover and simmer.
7. Taste and seasonbefore serving.
8. Serve warm Moroccan chicken with rice or couscous.
9. Garnish with fresh cilantro before serving.

NOTE:

➢ Add olives, preserved lemons, or chickpeasfor flavor and texture.
➢ In the final 30 minutes, To thicken the sauce, mix in 1 tablespoon cornstarch and 2 tablespoons water.
➢ Store leftovers for three to four days. Reheat gently in the microwave or stove before serving.

INGREDIENTS:

- ❖ 1 pound ground beef (or beef-pork combination)
- ❖ 1 onion, finely chopped
- ❖ 2 cloves garlic, minced
- ❖ 1 carrot, finely chopped
- ❖ 1 celery stalk, finely chopped
- ❖ 1 can (14 ounces) crushed tomatoes
- ❖ 1 can (6 ounces) tomato paste
- ❖ 1 cup beef broth
- ❖ 1/2 cup red wine (optional)
- ❖ 1 teaspoon dried oregano
- ❖ 1 teaspoon dried basil
- ❖ 1/2 teaspoon dried thyme
- ❖ Salt and pepper to taste
- ❖ 1 bay leaf
- ❖ 1 tablespoon olive oil
- ❖ Cooked spaghetti for serving
- ❖ Grated Parmesan cheese for serving
- ❖ Chopped fresh parsley for garnish (optional)

INSTRUCTIONS:

1. Pan-heat olive oil on medium. Spoon-break ground meat as it cooks.
2. Chopped onion, carrot, celery, and minced garlic in the skillet. Cook veggies for 5 minutes to tenderize.
3. Put steak and veggies in slow cooker.

4. In the slow cooker, add chopped tomatoes, tomato paste, beef broth, red wine (if desired), dried thyme, basil, oregano, salt, pepper, and bay leaf. Combine ingredients.
5. Stir regularly for 6–8 hours on low or 3–4 hours on high under cover.
6. Taste and season before serving.
7. To cook pasta al dente, follow package directions. Empty spaghetti.
8. Serve pasta with Bolognese.
9. Add chopped fresh parsley and grated Parmesan if preferred.

NOTE:

➤ You can alter this dish by adding extras to the sauce, such as olives, bell peppers, or mushrooms.
➤ The fridge can store leftover bolognese sauce for three to four days. Reheat gently in the microwave or stove before serving.

INGREDIENTS:

- ❖ 1 1/2 pounds beef sirloin steak, thinly sliced
- ❖ 1 onion, thinly sliced
- ❖ 8 ounces mushrooms, sliced
- ❖ 2 cloves garlic, minced
- ❖ 1 cup beef broth
- ❖ 2 tablespoons Worcestershire sauce
- ❖ 1 tablespoon Dijon mustard
- ❖ 1 teaspoon paprika
- ❖ Salt and pepper to taste
- ❖ 1 cup sour cream
- ❖ 2 tablespoons all-purpose flour
- ❖ Cooked egg noodles or rice for serving
- ❖ Chopped fresh parsley for garnish (optional)

INSTRUCTIONS:

1. The slow cooker should contain sliced beef sirloin steak, finely sliced onion, mushrooms, and minced garlic.
2. Mix beef broth, Worcestershire sauce, Dijon mustard, paprika, salt, and pepper in a bowl.
3. Cover the slow cooker beef and vegetables with broth. Mix well.
4. Cover and cook meat on low 6-8 hours or high 3-4 hours until tender.
5. Mix sour cream and all-purpose flour in a small bowl until smooth.
6. Mix the sour cream mixture into the slow cooker. Cover and simmer on low for 15–30 minutes to thicken the sauce.

7. Taste and season as needed.
8. Over egg noodles or rice, serve beef stroganoff.
9. Add chopped fresh parsley if desired.

NOTE:

➤ Add dry white wine or lemon juice for flavor.
➤ Last 30 minutes, add 1 spoonful of cornstarch and 2 teaspoons of water to the slow cooker to thicken the sauce.
➤ Refrigerated beef stroganoff lasts 3–4 days. Reheat gently on the burner or microwave before serving.

INGREDIENTS:

- ❖ 1-1/2 pounds boneless, skinless chicken breasts, diced
- ❖ 2 cups chicken broth
- ❖ 1 cup heavy cream
- ❖ 1/2 cup grated Parmesan cheese
- ❖ 1/4 cup unsalted butter, melted
- ❖ 3 cloves garlic, minced
- ❖ 1 teaspoon dried Italian seasoning
- ❖ Salt and pepper to taste
- ❖ 12 ounces of fettuccine or other pasta
- ❖ Chopped fresh parsley for garnish (optional)

INSTRUCTIONS:

1. Bite-sized chicken chunks, chicken broth, heavy cream, grated Parmesan cheese, melted unsalted butter, chopped garlic, dried Italian seasoning, salt, and pepper should all be combined in the slow cooker. Mix everything.
2. When the chicken is well cooked and soft, cover it and cook it for four to five hours on low or two to three hours on high.
3. Follow the package's instructions to cook the fettuccine for at least half an hour before serving. Remove the pasta's water.
4. Coat the cooked fettuccine in the creamy chicken Alfredo sauce by adding it to the slow cooker and stirring.
5. To ensure the flavors blend and the food is heated through, cover and cook for 15 to 30 minutes more on low heat.
6. If needed, adjust the seasoning by tasting it.

7. If preferred, top the hot chicken Alfredo with finely chopped fresh parsley.

NOTE:

- ➢ For added taste and texture, you can add additional items to the slow cooker in addition to the chicken, including sun-dried tomatoes or sliced mushrooms.
- ➢ You can smooth out an overly thick sauce by adding a little more chicken stock or heavy cream.
- ➢ Refrigerate leftovers for three to four days. Reheat gently in the microwave or stove before serving.

INGREDIENTS:

- ❖ 2 cups vegetable broth
- ❖ 1 can (14 ounces) diced tomatoes, undrained
- ❖ 2 carrots, peeled and sliced
- ❖ 2 potatoes, peeled and diced
- ❖ 1 onion, diced
- ❖ 2 cloves garlic, minced
- ❖ 1 cup sliced mushrooms
- ❖ 1 cup trimmed, bite-sized green beans
- ❖ 1 cup fresh and frozen or canned corn kernels
- ❖ 1 cup peas (fresh or frozen)
- ❖ 1 teaspoon dried thyme
- ❖ 1 teaspoon dried rosemary
- ❖ Salt and pepper to taste
- ❖ 2 tablespoons tomato paste (optional for extra richness)
- ❖ Chopped fresh parsley for garnish (optional)

INSTRUCTIONS:

1. Add the diced tomatoes and veggie broth to the slow cooker.
2. Chop onion, carrots, potatoes, and peas and put in slow cooker. Garlic, green beans, maize, and mushrooms should be added.
3. Stir in salt, pepper, dried thyme, and rosemary.
4. For added richness, mix in the tomato paste, if using.
5. Cover and simmer once the vegetables are soft for 6–8 hours on low or 3–4 hours on high.
6. If needed, adjust the seasoning by tasting it.

7. If preferred, top the hot vegetable stew with finely chopped fresh parsley.

NOTE:

- ➢ You can alter this vegetable stew by adding more veggies like bell peppers, squash, or celery, depending on your tastes.
- ➢ To add even more protein and fiber, feel free to add cooked beans or lentils.
- ➢ Leftovers can be frozen or refrigerated for three to four days. Reheat gently in the microwave or stove before serving.

INGREDIENTS:

For the pork:

- ❖ 1 1/2 pounds pork shoulder or pork loin, cut into bite-sized pieces
- ❖ 1/2 cup all-purpose flour
- ❖ Salt and pepper to taste
- ❖ 2 tablespoons vegetable oil

For the sauce:

- ❖ 1 cup pineapple juice
- ❖ 1/2 cup ketchup
- ❖ 1/4 cup brown sugar
- ❖ 1/4 cup apple cider vinegar
- ❖ 2 tablespoons soy sauce
- ❖ 1 teaspoon minced ginger
- ❖ 1 teaspoon minced garlic
- ❖ 1 bell pepper, diced
- ❖ 1 onion, diced
- ❖ 1 cup pineapple chunks (fresh or canned)

For thickening (optional):

- ❖ 2 tablespoons cornstarch
- ❖ 2 tablespoons water

INSTRUCTIONS:

1. Mix all-purpose flour, salt, and pepper in a shallow bowl. Dredge pork slices in flour mixture to coat evenly.
2. In a skillet, heat vegetable oil on medium-high. Heat the coated pork chunks for 4–5 minutes until browned. Put pork in a low-heat cooker.
3. Mix soy sauce, brown sugar, ketchup, apple cider vinegar, pineapple juice, and minced garlic and ginger in a large bowl.
4. Slow cooker meat should be covered in sauce. Mix in the diced onion, bell pepper, and pineapple.
5. Simmer covered for 6–8 hours on low or 3–4 hours on high after the meat is tender.
6. Make a cornstarch-water slurry in a small bowl to thicken the sauce. In the last 30 minutes of simmering, stir the slurry into the slow cooker
7. and season to taste.
8. Serve hot rice or noodles with sweet-and-sour pork.

NOTE:

➤ Other vegetables like carrots or snow peas
➤ can be added to the recipe.
➤ Add a splash of spicy sauce or red pepper flakes to spice up the sauce.
➤ Refrigerate leftovers for three to four days. Reheat gently in the microwave or stove before serving.

INGREDIENTS:

For the meatballs:

- ❖ 1 pound ground beef
- ❖ 1/2 cup breadcrumbs
- ❖ 1/4 cup grated Parmesan cheese
- ❖ One egg
- ❖ 2 cloves garlic, minced
- ❖ 1 teaspoon dried oregano
- ❖ 1 teaspoon dried basil
- ❖ Salt and pepper to taste

For the sauce:

- ❖ 1 can (28 ounces) crushed tomatoes
- ❖ 1 can (14 ounces) tomato sauce
- ❖ 1 onion, diced
- ❖ 2 cloves garlic, minced
- ❖ 1 teaspoon dried oregano
- ❖ 1 teaspoon dried basil
- ❖ Salt and pepper to taste

For assembling:

- ❖ Hoagie rolls or sub rolls
- ❖ Shredded mozzarella cheese
- ❖ Chopped fresh parsley (optional, for garnish)

INSTRUCTIONS:

1. Toss together the cooked ground beef, breadcrumbs, egg, grated Parmesan cheese, dried basil, dried oregano, salt, and pepper in a bulky bowl. Add each item one by one and mix until well combined.

2. Roll the meat mixture into meatballs, rolling each one to a diameter of approximately 1 to 1 1/2 inches.

3. Before placing in the slow cooker, combine the crushed tomatoes, tomato sauce, chopped onion, minced garlic, dried oregano, dried basil, salt, and pepper. Incorporate all ingredients.

4. Carefully drop the meatballs into the slow cooker's sauce mixture.

5. After 6–8 hours of low cooking or 3–4 hours of high cooking, the meatballs should be cooked through and soft. Cover and cook.

6. Before serving, set the oven to broil. After slicing the sub rolls or hoagie rolls lengthwise, lay them on a baking pan.

7. Put a little meatball and sauce on top of every roll. Add shredded mozzarella cheese on top.

8. Place the baking sheet under the broiler for one to two minutes or when the cheese is melted and bubbling.

9. Take it out of the oven and, if you like, top it with finely chopped fresh parsley.

10. If preferred, serve the meatball subs hot with more sauce for dipping.

NOTE:

- ➤ Meatball subs can be customized with a variety of toppings, including sliced mushrooms, sautéed onions and peppers, banana peppers, and more.
- ➤ If you make extra sauce and meatballs, you can store them in the fridge for up to four days. Warm it up little in the oven or microwave before serving.

33. BLACK BEAN SOUP

INGREDIENTS:

- ❖ Two fifteen-ounce cans of black beans that have been rinsed and drained
- ❖ 1 onion, diced
- ❖ 2 cloves garlic, minced
- ❖ 1 bell pepper, diced (any color)
- ❖ 1 jalapeño pepper, seeded and diced (optional, for heat)
- ❖ 1 carrot, diced
- ❖ 1 stalk celery, diced
- ❖ 1 can (14 ounces) diced tomatoes, undrained
- ❖ 4 cups vegetable broth
- ❖ 1 teaspoon ground cumin
- ❖ 1 teaspoon chili powder
- ❖ 1/2 teaspoon smoked paprika
- ❖ Salt and pepper to taste
- ❖ Juice of 1 lime
- ❖ Chopped fresh cilantro for garnish
- ❖ Toppings like sour cream or Greek yogurt can be added before serving.
- ❖ Avocado, sliced (if desired)

INSTRUCTIONS:

1. The slow cooker should be stocked with the following ingredients: garlic, onion, bell pepper, jalapeño pepper, carrot, celery, tomatoes, vegetable broth, ground cumin, chili powder, smoked paprika, salt, and pepper. Mix everything together.

2. Cover and simmer for 6-8 hours on low heat or 3-4 hours on high heat until the vegetables are soft and the flavors have combined.
3. To achieve a smooth consistency, purée the soup using an immersion blender. As an alternative, you might mix some of the soup until it's smooth, and then put it back in the slow cooker.
4. Combine the lime juice with the other ingredients.
5. To determine if the seasoning needs to be adjusted, you can give it a taste.
6. In a separate bowl, spoon some black bean soup. Chopped cilantro can be added on top for aesthetic reasons.
7. Top with sliced avocado and, if desired, a dollop of sour cream or Greek yogurt. Hot is best.

NOTE:

➢ For added texture to the soup, you can reserve a few black beans before blending and add them in.
➢ Any extra soup, when stored in an airtight container, can be frozen for later use. Yes, it freezes solid. Warm it up a little in the oven or microwave before serving.
➢ Soup toppings like shredded cheese, chopped red onion, or a spritz of fresh lime juice are totally up to you.

INGREDIENTS:

- ❖ 4 boneless, skinless chicken breasts
- ❖ Salt and pepper to taste
- ❖ 1/2 cup all-purpose flour
- ❖ 2 tablespoons olive oil
- ❖ 4 tablespoons butter
- ❖ 1 cup sliced mushrooms
- ❖ 1/2 cup Marsala wine
- ❖ 1/2 cup chicken broth
- ❖ 1/2 cup heavy cream
- ❖ 2 tablespoons chopped fresh parsley (for garnish)

INSTRUCTIONS:

1. Coat the chicken breasts in flour, making sure to shake off any excess, after seasoning them with salt and pepper.
2. In a large skillet, melt the butter and olive oil over medium-high heat.
3. After the pan is heated, sear the chicken breasts for approximately 5 minutes per side, or until they develop a golden brown hue. Remove the chicken from the pan before placing it aside.
4. Coat the mushrooms by adding them to the pan with the reserved 2 tablespoons of butter and stirring to combine. Toss the mushrooms into the sauté pan when they are soft and have browned somewhat.
5. After brown bits have been scraped off the bottom of the skillet, stir in the chicken broth and Marsala wine.

6. Cook, stirring occasionally, for five minutes at a low simmer to reduce sauce thickness.
7. Return the chicken breasts to the skillet after adding the heavy cream and stirring.
8. Ten further minutes of simmering should be enough time for the chicken to cook through and for the sauce to thicken.
9. Sprinkle chopped parsley on top before serving.

NOTE:

➢ Traditionally, mashed potatoes or noodles are served with chicken marsala along with a side salad.
➢ If you want a more decadent sauce, toss a tablespoon of cornstarch and cold water in the final few minutes of simmering.
➢ If the chicken breasts are overcooked, they can turn dry, so proceed with caution. Adjust the cooking time as necessary, depending on their thickness.

35. THAI GREEN CURRY

INGREDIENTS:

- ❖ Chicken breasts or thighs, skinless and boneless, weighing 1 pound, diced into bite-sized pieces
- ❖ Salt and pepper to taste
- ❖ 2 tablespoons vegetable oil
- ❖ 2-3 tablespoons green curry paste
- ❖ 1 can (13.5 ounces) coconut milk
- ❖ 1 cup chicken broth
- ❖ 2 tablespoons fish sauce
- ❖ 1 tablespoon brown sugar
- ❖ 1 bell pepper, thinly sliced
- ❖ 1 small eggplant, diced
- ❖ 1 cup green beans, trimmed and halved
- ❖ 1 cup sliced bamboo shoots (optional)
- ❖ Tear 1 cup of fresh basil leaves (tame basil leaves, normal basil, or Thai basil)
- ❖ Cooked jasmine rice for serving

INSTRUCTIONS:

1. Season the chicken with salt and pepper.
2. In a big wok or pan, heat the vegetable oil over medium heat.
3. Put the green curry paste in the pan when it begins to smell good and stir-fry it for a minute or two.
4. Combine all the ingredients after adding the coconut milk and chicken broth.
5. Toss in the fish sauce and brown sugar, stirring to dissolve the sugar.

6. To the skillet, add the sliced bell pepper, green beans, eggplant, and, if desired, the bamboo shoots. Blend all of the ingredients.
7. Once the chicken is done and the vegetables are soft, reduce the heat and simmer for 10 to 15 minutes.
8. You can add more sugar, fish sauce, salt, or pepper after you taste
9. the curry to make it taste exactly right.
10. Add the Thai basil leaves that have been split up and sauté for another minute.
11. Jasmine rice, once cooked, goes well with hot Thai green curry.

NOTE:

- ➢ The spice level in green curry paste varies, so adapt the amount to your preferred heat level.
- ➢ You can alter the vegetables in the curry to suit your tastes or what you have on hand. Carrots, mushrooms, and zucchini are additional veggies that taste good in Thai green curry.
- ➢ Thai basil gives the curry a unique flavor, but standard basil will substitute if you need help finding Thai basil.
- ➢ Curry leftovers, if sealed in a container, can keep for three days in the fridge. Return to a low heat and cook for a few more minutes before serving.

36. MUSHROOM RISOTTO

INGREDIENTS:

- ❖ 1 1/2 cups Arborio rice
- ❖ 6 cups chicken or vegetable broth
- ❖ 2 tablespoons olive oil
- ❖ 1 onion, finely chopped
- ❖ 2 cloves garlic, minced
- ❖ Mushrooms (cremini or button)—1 pound, sliced
- ❖ 1/2 cup dry white wine (optional)
- ❖ 1/2 cup grated Parmesan cheese
- ❖ 2 tablespoons butter
- ❖ Salt and pepper to taste
- ❖ Chopped fresh parsley for garnish

INSTRUCTIONS:

1. Whether you're cooking chicken or vegetables, the best way to make broth is to simmer it over medium heat. Keep the risotto covered and cooked over medium heat.
2. In a big Dutch oven or skillet, bring the olive oil to a shimmer. The chopped onion should be tender after an additional three or four minutes of boiling.
3. After a minute or two of boiling, add the minced garlic and keep cooking until it starts to exude a pleasant aroma.
4. After the mushrooms' liquid has evaporated and the slices have acquired a golden brown
5. hue, remove them from the pan and continue sautéing for an additional 6 to 8 minutes.
6. For the first minute or two of cooking, toss the Arborio rice often until it starts to turn a little brown.

7. After the white wine has evaporated, reduce heat to low and simmer, stirring frequently.
8. Ladle in the boiling broth while stirring continuously. Continue adding broth until the rice has absorbed a portion. The ideal texture for cooked rice is a somewhat hard inside and a soft, creamy outside; this should be achieved after 20 to 25 minutes.
9. Take the risotto off the fire and stir in the butter and grated Parmesan after it has thickened to your liking. Season to taste with salt and pepper.
10. Garnish the cooked mushroom risotto with some finely chopped parsley right before serving.

NOTE:

➢ Risotto needs to be constantly stirred and watched to get a creamy texture, so be ready to spend much time near the stove while it cooks.
➢ with a vegetarian option, you can substitute vegetable broth with the chicken stock.
➢ You may easily alter this dish by adding extras like peas, spinach, or roasted garlic for more taste.
➢ Risotto leftovers can be stored in an airtight container for up to three days in the refrigerator. If necessary, loosen the mixture with a splash of water or broth during the gentle reheating process on the stovetop or in the microwave.

INGREDIENTS:

- ❖ 1 lb (450g) ground beef
- ❖ 1 onion, chopped
- ❖ 2 cloves garlic, minced
- ❖ 1 can (14.5 oz) diced tomatoes, undrained
- ❖ 1 can (15 oz) tomato sauce
- ❖ 1 can (15 oz) kidney beans, drained and rinsed
- ❖ 1 can (4 oz) diced green chilies
- ❖ 2 cups (475 ml) beef broth
- ❖ 1 tablespoon chili powder
- ❖ 1 teaspoon ground cumin
- ❖ 1 teaspoon paprika
- ❖ Salt and pepper to taste
- ❖ 2 cups (200g) uncooked elbow macaroni
- ❖ 1 cup (120g) shredded cheddar cheese
- ❖ Optional toppings: chopped green onions, sour cream, additional shredded cheese

INSTRUCTIONS:

1. The ground beef should be cooked in a big skillet over medium-high heat. Remove any extra fat.
2. When the onion is tender, sauté it for two to three minutes more in the skillet with the ground beef after adding the chopped onion and minced garlic.
3. Add the garlic, onion, and cooked beef to the slow cooker.
4. Chop the tomatoes and kidney beans and throw them into the slow cooker with the diced green chilies, tomato sauce,

chili powder, cumin, paprika, salt, and pepper. Thoroughly combine all ingredients.

5. Cook, covered, for 6–8 hours on low heat or 3–4 hours on high heat.
6. Before serving, mix in the uncooked elbow macaroni. Once the macaroni is soft, continue cooking it covered.
7. When the macaroni is cooked, add the shredded cheddar cheese and toss until it melts and is thoroughly mixed.
8. Serve hot, with more shredded cheese, sour cream, or chopped green onions as optional garnishes.

NOTE:

➢ To achieve the desired level of heat in the chili mac, simply adjust the quantity of chili powder and chopped green chilies
➢ to your liking.
➢ Refrigerate any leftovers for no more than three days if sealed tightly. Warm it up little in the oven or microwave before serving.

INGREDIENTS:

- ❖ 1 lb (450g) dried navy beans, rinsed and soaked overnight
- ❖ 1 ham hock or 1 cup diced ham
- ❖ 1 onion, chopped
- ❖ 2 carrots, peeled and chopped
- ❖ 2 celery stalks, chopped
- ❖ 2 cloves garlic, minced
- ❖ 6 cups (1.4 liters) chicken or vegetable broth
- ❖ 2 bay leaves
- ❖ 1 teaspoon dried thyme
- ❖ Salt and pepper to taste
- ❖ Chopped fresh parsley for garnish (optional)

INSTRUCTIONS:

1. Put the navy beans in the slow cooker after draining.
2. Arrange chopped ham or ham hock atop the beans.
3. Toss in the chopped carrots, celery, onion, and garlic once the slow cooker is hot.
4. After adding the broth to the slow cooker, mix to combine (you can use chicken or vegetable broth).
5. Before adding the dried bay leaves and thyme, gather them.
6. Season to taste with salt and pepper.
7. Gently combine all the ingredients.
8. Once the beans have softened and the flavors have blended, cover and simmer for 8-10 hours on low heat (or 4-6 hours on high).
9. After soup has cooked, t

10. ake the ham hock out of the slow cooker. If you have any leftover ham hock, shred it and throw it in the soup. The extra fat and bone should be disposed of.
11. Before you add any seasoning, give the soup a taste.
12. For an extra flavor punch, sprinkle the cooked dish with some freshly chopped parsley.

NOTE:

➤ Use an immersion blender to purée some of the vegetables and beans, or mash some with a fork, to make a heartier soup.
➤ The flavors in this soup continue to combine the next day, making it even delicious. Leftovers, if sealed in a glass container, will keep for up to three days in the refrigerator. Just give it a quick reheat in the oven or microwave before you serve it.

INGREDIENTS:

- ❖ Chicken thighs, skinless and boneless, 1 pound (450 grams), diced into bite-sized portions
- ❖ Andouille or kielbasa, or other smoked sausages, sliced, 1 pound (450 grams)
- ❖ 1 onion, chopped
- ❖ 1 bell pepper, chopped
- ❖ 2 celery stalks, chopped
- ❖ 3 cloves garlic, minced
- ❖ 1 can (14.5 oz) diced tomatoes, undrained
- ❖ 4 cups (946ml) chicken broth
- ❖ 1/4 cup (60ml) vegetable oil or melted butter
- ❖ 1/4 cup (30g) all-purpose flour
- ❖ 2 bay leaves
- ❖ 1 teaspoon dried thyme
- ❖ 1 teaspoon dried oregano
- ❖ 1 teaspoon paprika
- ❖ 1/2 teaspoon cayenne pepper (adjust to taste)
- ❖ Salt and pepper to taste
- ❖ Cooked white rice for serving
- ❖ Chopped green onions and parsley for garnish

INSTRUCTIONS:

1. In a big skillet, melt the butter or vegetable oil over medium heat. To make a roux, mix the flour and water together. The roux should become a rich brown color after simmering for 10 to 15 minutes with constant stirring. Make sure not to burn it.
2. To thicken the roux, add it to a saucepan and simmer it over low heat.
3. Season with salt and pepper after dicing the red onion, green pepper, celery, garlic, tomatoes, chicken broth, paprika, oregano, cayenne pepper, bay leaves, thyme, and
4. chicken
5. broth. Toss the
6. ingredients to combine.

NOTE:

➢ Although cornbread or crusty bread is good with gumbo, rice is the traditional serving vessel.
➢ To enhance the flavor, fry the sausage slices on a skillet prior to placing them in the slow cooker.
➢ Using shrimp or other seafood is a simple way to change this dish. Putting them in the slow cooker for the last half an hour is all that's required.

INGREDIENTS:

- ❖ Deveined and peeled big shrimp weighing 1 pound (450 grams)
- ❖ 1 onion, chopped
- ❖ 1 bell pepper, chopped
- ❖ 2 celery stalks, chopped
- ❖ 3 cloves garlic, minced
- ❖ 1 can (14.5 oz) diced tomatoes, undrained
- ❖ 1 can (8 oz) tomato sauce
- ❖ 1 cup (240ml) chicken broth
- ❖ 2 tablespoons tomato paste
- ❖ 1 tablespoon Worcestershire sauce
- ❖ 1 teaspoon dried thyme
- ❖ 1 teaspoon dried oregano
- ❖ 1 teaspoon paprika
- ❖ 1/4 teaspoon cayenne pepper (adjust to taste)
- ❖ Salt and pepper to taste
- ❖ Cooked white rice, for serving
- ❖ Chopped fresh parsley for garnish

INSTRUCTIONS:

1. Add the chopped onion, bell pepper, celery, minced garlic, diced tomatoes, tomato paste, Worcestershire sauce, chicken broth, oregano, paprika, cayenne pepper, salt, and pepper to the slow cooker. Mix everything until thoroughly mixed.

2. Cover, reduce heat, and simmer for 6–8 hours on low or 3–4 hours on high, or until the veggies are soft and the flavors have combined.
3. Stir in the peeled and deveined shrimp 15 to 20 minutes before serving. Once the shrimp are pink and thoroughly cooked, cover and continue cooking.
4. If required, taste the shrimp creole and adjust the seasoning.
5. Serve hot cooked white rice with chopped fresh parsley as a garnish.

NOTE:

➢ While shrimp creole is typically served over rice, it's equally delicious over cornbread or crusty toast.
➢ To achieve a thicker sauce, combine one tablespoon of cornstarch with two teaspoons of water and add it to the slow cooker in the final half-hour of cooking.
➢ To su
➢ To your taste, feel free to add more or less cayenne pepper to change the amount of heat.
➢ The leftovers will remain fresh for at least two days if sealed in a container and refrigerated. Just give it a quick reheat in the oven or microwave before you serve it.

Ingredients:

- ❖ 2 lbs (900g) lamb shoulder or beef chuck, cut into bite-sized pieces
- ❖ 4 large potatoes, peeled and diced
- ❖ 3 carrots, peeled and sliced
- ❖ 2 onions, chopped
- ❖ 2 cloves garlic, minced
- ❖ 4 cups (946ml) beef or vegetable broth
- ❖ 2 tablespoons tomato paste
- ❖ 1 tablespoon Worcestershire sauce
- ❖ 1 teaspoon dried thyme
- ❖ 1 teaspoon dried rosemary
- ❖ Salt and pepper to taste
- ❖ Chopped fresh parsley for garnish (optional)

INSTRUCTIONS:

1. Pour some oil into a big skillet and set it over medium-high heat. After approximately 5 minutes, add the diced beef or lamb and heat until browned on all sides.Make sure to sear the meat before adding it to the slow cooker.
2. Toss in the potatoes, carrots, onions, and garlic to the slow cooker.
3. For a well-integrated sauce, whisk together Worcestershire sauce, dried thyme, rosemary, salt, pepper, tomato paste, and beef or vegetable stock. After you've mixed everything, place it in the slow cooker.
4. Thoroughly combine all of the ingredients.

5. Meat and veggies can be cooked to perfection by simmering covered over low heat for 6-8 hours or high heat for 3-4 hours
6. .
7. If you think the stew might need more seasoning, give it a taste.
8. Arrange in a preheated casserole and, if like, top with finely chopped parsley.

NOTE:

➢ Although lamb is a common ingredient in traditional Irish stew, beef is a good replacement.
➢ The vegetables can be tailored to suit your personal taste. Another typical ingredient in Irish stew
➢ is turnips or parsnips.
➢ You can keep leftovers in the fridge for up to three days if you seal them in a container. Warm through, stirring occasionally, in a microwave or skillet, just until serving time.

42. SLOW COOKER CHICKEN AND SAUSAGE JAMBALAYA

INGREDIENTS:

- ❖ Chicken thighs, skinless and boneless, 1 pound (450 grams), diced into bite-sized portions
- ❖ Sliced smoked sausage (e.g., andouille or kielbasa), 1 pound (450 grams)
- ❖ 1 onion, chopped
- ❖ 1 bell pepper, chopped
- ❖ 2 celery stalks, chopped
- ❖ 3 cloves garlic, minced
- ❖ 1 can (14.5 oz) diced tomatoes, undrained
- ❖ 1 cup (240ml) chicken broth
- ❖ 1 cup (200g) long-grain white rice
- ❖ 2 teaspoons Cajun seasoning
- ❖ 1 teaspoon dried thyme
- ❖ 1 teaspoon dried oregano
- ❖ 1/2 teaspoon paprika
- ❖ 1/4 teaspoon cayenne pepper (adjust to taste)
- ❖ Salt and pepper to taste
- ❖ Chopped fresh parsley for garnish

INSTRUCTIONS:

1. Add the rice, diced tomatoes, Cajun seasoning, paprika, oregano, cayenne pepper, salt, pepper, and minced garlic to a slow cooker. Bring to a simmer. Simmer, stirring occasionally, for a few hours over low heat. Gently incorporate the chopped tomatoes, peppers, celery, and onion. Toss the ingredients together until they are well blended.
2. Add the diced chicken thighs and sliced smoked sausage to the slow cooker. Stir to ensure even distribution.
3. Once the rice is soft, the sausage is heated, and the chicken is thoroughly cooked, cover and simmer on low heat for 6–8 hours or on high heat for 3–4 hours.
4. After the jambalaya is cooked, taste it and adjust the seasoning if needed.
5. Serve hot, with freshly chopped parsley as a garnish.

NOTE:

➢ To give this jambalaya a more typical Creole flavor, you can add other ingredients like shrimp, chopped tomatoes with green chilies, or okra.
➢ To suit your taste, add or subtract cayenne pepper and Cajun seasoning to change the heat.
➢ The shelf life of leftovers in the fridge is extended by three days when sealed in an airtight container. Return to a low heat and cook for a few more minutes before serving.

INGREDIENTS:

- ❖ 1 (3-4 lb) corned beef brisket with spice packet
- ❖ 6 red potatoes, quartered
- ❖ 4 carrots, cut into 2-inch pieces
- ❖ 1 onion, peeled and cut into wedges
- ❖ 1 small head of cabbage, cut into wedges
- ❖ 4 cups (946ml) water (or enough to cover the corned beef)
- ❖ 1 cup (240ml) beef broth
- ❖ 2 bay leaves
- ❖ 1 teaspoon whole black peppercorns
- ❖ 1 teaspoon mustard seeds
- ❖ Optional: whole cloves

INSTRUCTIONS:

1. Use paper towels to gently dry the corned beef brisket after giving it a quick rinse in cold water.
2. Put the red potatoes, quartered, in the slow cooker's bottom.
3. With the fat side facing up, place the corned beef brisket atop the potatoes.
4. Over the brisket, scatter the spice packet, which is included with the corned beef.
5. Around the brisket in the slow cooker, arrange the onion wedges and carrot slices.
6. Add the mustard seeds, bay leaves, whole black peppercorns, and, if desired, whole cloves to the slow cooker.

7. After the brisket is almost coated, pour the water and beef broth.
8. Slowly cook, covered, for 8–10 hours or until fork-tender, or sear, uncovered, for 4–6 hours over high heat.
9. About one hour before serving, place the brisket in the slow cooker with the wedges of cabbage. Gently cook the cabbage until it becomes tender without being mushy.
10. Let the brisket rest for a few minutes after removing it from the slow cooker, and then slice it thinly against the grain.
11. Serve the corned beef slices with the cooked vegetables and a ladleful of the cooking liquid.

NOTE:

> ➢ You can divide the brisket in half and arrange the halves side by side in the slow cooker if they are too small to fit the whole brisket.
> ➢ You can alter the flavor by adding extra spices or herbs, such as garlic, thyme, or rosemary.
> ➢ Refrigerate leftovers in an airtight jar for three days. Reheat gently in the microwave or stove before serving.

44. SLOW COOKER TURKEY CHILI

INGREDIENTS:

- ❖ 1 lb (450g) ground turkey
- ❖ 1 onion, chopped
- ❖ 1 bell pepper, chopped
- ❖ 2 cloves garlic, minced
- ❖ 1 can (14.5 oz) diced tomatoes, undrained
- ❖ 1 can (15 oz) tomato sauce
- ❖ 1 can (15 oz) kidney beans, drained and rinsed
- ❖ 1 can (4 oz) diced green chilies
- ❖ 1 cup (240ml) chicken broth
- ❖ 2 tablespoons tomato paste
- ❖ 1 tablespoon chili powder
- ❖ 1 teaspoon ground cumin
- ❖ 1 teaspoon paprika
- ❖ 1/2 teaspoon dried oregano
- ❖ Salt and pepper to taste
- ❖ Optional toppings: shredded cheese, sour cream, chopped green onions, diced avocado

INSTRUCTIONS:

1. While browning ground turkey in a large skillet over medium-high heat, break it up with a spoon. Remove excess fat.
2. After cooking, transfer the turkey to the slow cooker.
3. Add the diced tomatoes, kidney beans, chopped green chilies, chopped onion, bell pepper, minced garlic, tomato sauce, tomato paste, chili powder, cumin, paprika,

oregano, salt, and pepper to the slow cooker. Mix everything until thoroughly mixed.

4. Cover and cook on low for 6–8 hours or high for 3–4 hours until the chili thickens and flavors mix.
5. If needed, taste the chili and adjust the seasoning.
6. Serve hot, topped with your preferred toppings (diced avocado, chopped green onions, sour cream, or shredded cheese).

NOTE:

➢ You can change this chili by adding chopped tomatoes with green chilies, black beans, or corn.
➢ Refrigerate leftovers in an airtight jar for three days. Reheat gently in the microwave or stove before serving.

INGREDIENTS:

For the filling:

- ❖ 1 lb (450g) ground beef or lamb
- ❖ 1 onion, chopped
- ❖ 2 carrots, diced
- ❖ 2 cloves garlic, minced
- ❖ 1 cup (150g) frozen peas
- ❖ 1 cup (240ml) beef broth
- ❖ 2 tablespoons tomato paste
- ❖ 1 tablespoon Worcestershire sauce
- ❖ 1 teaspoon dried thyme
- ❖ 1 teaspoon dried rosemary
- ❖ Salt and pepper to taste
- ❖ 2 tablespoons all-purpose flour (optional for thickening)

For the mashed potatoes:

- ❖ 2 lbs (900g) potatoes, peeled and diced
- ❖ 4 tablespoons butter
- ❖ 1/2 cup (120ml) milk
- ❖ Salt and pepper to taste
- ❖ 1 cup (100g) shredded cheddar cheese (optional for topping)

INSTRUCTIONS:

1. Break up ground beef or lamb with a spoon while it browns in a large skillet over medium-high heat. Remove excess fat.
2. Put prepared meat in slow cooker.
3. In the slow cooker, add diced carrots, onion, garlic, frozen peas, tomato paste, beef broth, Worcestershire sauce, dried thyme, rosemary, salt, and pepper. Thoroughly combine everything.
4. Cover and simmer 6-8 hours on low or 3-4 hours on high until filling is done and flavors mix.
5. For a richer filling, slurry 2 tablespoons all-purpose flour with water 30 minutes before serving and stir it into the filling. Heat another 30 minutes to thicken.
6. Make the mashed potatoes one hour before serving. Boil chopped potatoes in salted water. Simmer 15–20 minutes until potatoes are fork-tender. Return potatoes to pot after draining.
7. When potatoes are creamy, mash them with butter and milk. Season with salt and pepper to taste.
8. Smooth the mashed potatoes over the slow cooker, filling with a spatula.
9. If desired, add shredded cheddar cheese to mashed potatoes.
10. After 30 minutes, cover and simmer on high until cheese melts and mashed potatoes are warm.
11. Eat your delicious Shepherd's Pie hot!

NOTE:

- ➢ You can add maize or green beans to the stuffing.
- ➢ Refrigerate leftovers in an airtight jar for three days. Reheat gently in the microwave or stove before serving.

46. SLOW COOKER CHICKEN ENCHILADA SOUP

INGREDIENTS:

- ❖ 1 lb (450g) boneless, skinless chicken breasts
- ❖ 1 onion, chopped
- ❖ 2 cloves garlic, minced
- ❖ 1 can (14.5 oz) diced tomatoes, undrained
- ❖ 1 can (10 oz) red enchilada sauce
- ❖ 1 can (4 oz) diced green chilies
- ❖ one can (15 oz) of rinsed and drained black beans
- ❖ 240ml chicken broth
- ❖ 1 teaspoon ground cumin
- ❖ 1 teaspoon chili powder
- ❖ 1/2 teaspoon dried oregano
- ❖ Salt and pepper to taste
- ❖ 1 cup (120g) frozen corn kernels
- ❖ 1/4 cup (60ml) heavy cream or sour cream (optional, for added creaminess)
- ❖ Tortilla chips, shredded cheese, chopped cilantro, lime wedges for serving

INSTRUCTIONS:

1. Place chicken breasts in slow cooker.
2. In the slow cooker, add diced tomatoes, onion, garlic, red enchilada sauce, green chilies, black beans, chicken broth, ground cumin, chili powder, dried oregano, salt, and pepper.
3. Thoroughly combine everything.
4. Cover and stew the chicken for 6–8 hours on low or 3–4 hours on high when it is tender.

5. Shred the slow-cooked chicken breasts with two forks 30 minutes before serving. Slow-cook chicken scraps again.
6. Stir in frozen corn kernels and sour or heavy cream. Simmer the soup for 30 minutes to heat and thicken.
7. Taste and season soup as needed.
8. Lime wedges, cilantro, shredded cheese, and tortilla chips garnish hot dish.

NOTE:

➢ Change the amount of diced green chilies, chili powder, and mild or spicy enchilada sauce to customize the heat.
➢ Customize your dish with diced tomatoes, avocado, or jalapenos.
➢ Refrigerate leftovers in an airtight jar for three days. Reheat gently in the microwave or stove before serving.

47. SLOW COOKER BRAISED SHORT RIBS

INGREDIENTS:

- ❖ 4 lbs (1.8 kg) beef short ribs, bone-in
- ❖ Salt and pepper to taste
- ❖ 2 tablespoons olive oil
- ❖ 1 onion, chopped
- ❖ 2 carrots, chopped
- ❖ 2 celery stalks, chopped
- ❖ 4 cloves garlic, minced
- ❖ 1 cup (240ml) beef broth
- ❖ 1 cup (240ml) red wine (such as Cabernet Sauvignon or Merlot)
- ❖ 2 tablespoons tomato paste
- ❖ 2 tablespoons Worcestershire sauce
- ❖ 2 sprigs fresh thyme
- ❖ 2 sprigs fresh rosemary
- ❖ 2 bay leaves
- ❖ 1 tablespoon cornstarch (optional for thickening)

INSTRUCTIONS:

1. Spice up your short ribs with plenty of salt and pepper.
2. With the heat set to medium-high, warm the olive oil in a big skillet. Sear the short ribs for three to four minutes per side after turning them over. Slowly sauté the short ribs.
3. Add diced onion, celery, carrots, and minced garlic to the skillet. Cook vegetables for 5 minutes, stirring regularly, until tender.
4. Add short ribs and cooked vegetables to the slow cooker.

5. Bowl together tomato paste, red wine, Worcestershire sauce, and beef broth. Stir mixture into slow cooker with short ribs and veggies.
6. Add fresh thyme, rosemary, and bay leaves to the slow cooker.
7. Cover th
8. e short ribs and simmer for 8–10 hours on low or 4–6 hours on high until tender and falling off the bone.
9. Serve short ribs in a dish. Foil them for warmth.
10. Stir one tablespoon of cornstarch into one cup of water to thicken sauce. Simmer the slurry on high for 15–20 minutes in the slow cooker to thicken.Cover cooked and heated short ribs with sauce and vegetables.

NOTE:

➢ Braised short ribs go well with mashed potatoes, polenta, or risotto.
➢ Leftover meals should be refrigerated in an airtight jar for three days. Reheat food slowly in the microwave or stovetop before serving.

INGREDIENTS:

- 1 cup (200g) dried cannellini beans, soaked overnight and drained
- 1 onion, chopped
- Two carrots, peeled and chopped
- 2 celery stalks, chopped
- 3 cloves garlic, minced
- 4 cups (946ml) chicken or vegetable broth
- 1 can (14.5 oz) diced tomatoes, undrained
- 1 teaspoon dried thyme
- 1 teaspoon dried rosemary
- 1 teaspoon dried oregano
- Salt and pepper to taste
- 2 cups (60g) fresh spinach leaves, chopped
- 1/4 cup (60ml) heavy cream or half-and-half (optional)
- Grated Parmesan cheese for serving
- Crusty bread for serving

INSTRUCTIONS:

1. Soak cannellini beans, then add chopped onion, carrots, celery, minced garlic, diced tomatoes, chicken or vegetable broth, dried thyme, rosemary, oregano, salt, and pepper to the slow cooker. Thoroughly combine everything.
2. After the beans are tender, cover and cook for 8–10 hours on low or 4–6 hours on high.
3. Add chopped fresh spinach and heavy cream or half-and-half 30 minutes before serving. To reheat and soften spinach

4. , boil the soup for 30 minutes.
5. Taste and season soup as needed.
6. Serve the dish warm with crispy bread and freshly grated Parmesan cheese.

NOTE:

➢ You may change this soup by adding different veggies, including chopped kale or diced zucchini.
➢ Before adding the chopped onion, carrots, celery, and garlic to the slow cooker, you can sauté them in a skillet with a little olive oil for extra flavor.
➢ Refrigerate leftovers in an airtight jar for three days. Reheat gently in the microwave or stove before serving.

INGREDIENTS:

For the broth:

- ❖ 2 lbs (900g) chicken thighs, bone-in and skin-on
- ❖ 1 onion, halved
- ❖ 3-inch piece of ginger, sliced
- ❖ 4 cloves garlic, smashed
- ❖ 2 cinnamon sticks
- ❖ 4-star anise
- ❖ 6 cups (1.4 liters) chicken broth
- ❖ 2 cups (470ml) water
- ❖ 2 tablespoons fish sauce
- ❖ 1 tablespoon soy sauce
- ❖ 1 tablespoon sugar
- ❖ Salt, to taste
- ❖ For the soup:
- ❖ 8 oz (225g) rice noodles (banh pho)
- ❖ Cooked chicken meat from the thighs, shredded
- ❖ 1 onion, thinly sliced
- ❖ 2 cups (120g) bean sprouts
- ❖ Fresh cilantro leaves
- ❖ Fresh Thai basil leaves
- ❖ Lime wedges
- ❖ Sriracha sauce (optional)
- ❖ Hoisin sauce (optional)

INSTRUCTIONS:

1. In a large slow cooker, combine chicken thighs, water, fish sauce, soy sauce, sugar, salt, cinnamon sticks, sliced ginger, smashed garlic, half onion, star anise, and chicken stock.
2. Cover and stew the chicken for 6–8 hours on low or 3–4 hours on high when it is tender.
3. Remove the slow-cooked chicken thighs and shred with two forks after the soup is done. Discard skin and bones.
4. Pour the broth into a different pot after straining it through cheesecloth or a fine-mesh screen, throwing away the solids.
5. As directed on the package, cook the rice noodles. After draining, set away.
6. Spoon cooked rice noodles into dishes to serve. Add the bean sprouts, thinly sliced onion, and shredded chicken.
7. Pour the steaming broth over the chicken and noodles.
8. Serve hot with fresh cilantro, Thai basil, lime wedges, and, for personalization, Sriracha and hoisin sauces on the side.

NOTE:

➢ Feel free to add extra toppings to your pho, including thinly sliced Thai chiles, chopped green onions, or sliced jalapeños.
➢ If you want the broth to be clearer before serving, you can skim any extra fat from its surface.
➢ You can refrigerate the leftover broth and chicken separately for up to three days. Before serving, slowly reheat over the stove. Toppings and noodles should be kept apart in storage and added right before serving.

INGREDIENTS:

- ❖ 2 lbs (900g) beef chuck roast, trimmed of excess fat and cut into large chunks
- ❖ Salt and pepper to taste
- ❖ 2 tablespoons olive oil
- ❖ 1 onion, finely chopped
- ❖ 2 carrots, diced
- ❖ 2 celery stalks, diced
- ❖ 4 cloves garlic, minced
- ❖ 1 can (14.5 oz) crushed tomatoes
- ❖ 1 can (6 oz) tomato paste
- ❖ 1 cup (240ml) beef broth
- ❖ 1/2 cup (120ml) red wine (optional)
- ❖ 2 bay leaves
- ❖ 1 teaspoon dried thyme
- ❖ 1 teaspoon dried oregano
- ❖ 1 teaspoon dried rosemary
- ❖ 1/2 teaspoon red pepper flakes (optional)
- ❖ Cooked pasta for serving
- ❖ Grated Parmesan cheese for serving
- ❖ Fresh chopped parsley, for garnish

INSTRUCTIONS:

1. Season pork cubes on all sides with salt and pepper.
2. Get a big pan hot and add the olive oil. It takes three to four minutes per side to brown the beef cubes. After browning the steak, slowly boil it.

3. Add minced garlic, carrots, celery, and diced onion to the skillet. Simmer 5 minutes, stirring occasionally, until vegetables are tender.
4. Mix beef and vegetables in the slow cooker.
5. In the slow cooker, add crushed tomatoes, tomato paste, beef broth, red wine (if used), bay leaves, dried thyme, oregano, rosemary, and red pepper flakes. Thoroughly combine everything.
6. The meat should be fork-tender and come apart after 8–10 hours of moderate heat or 4–6 hours of high heat under a cover.
7. Throw away the slow cooker bay leaves after cooking.
8. Fork-shred meat and sauce in the slow cooker.
9. Before serving the meat ragu, sprinkle grated Parmesan and fresh parsley on the spaghetti.

NOTE:

➤ Beef ragu goes with penne, fettuccine, or spaghetti.
➤ Refrigerate leftovers in an airtight jar for three days. Reheat gently in the microwave or stove before serving.

INGREDIENTS

- ❖ 1 ½ pounds chunked boneless, skinless chicken breasts or thighs
- ❖ 4 cups chicken broth
- ❖ 2 cups frozen peas and carrots mix
- ❖ 1 cup frozen corn
- ❖ 3 medium potatoes, peeled and diced
- ❖ 1 large onion, chopped
- ❖ 3 garlic cloves, minced
- ❖ 1 cup heavy cream
- ❖ ⅓ cup all-purpose flour
- ❖ 2 teaspoons dried thyme
- ❖ 1 teaspoon dried rosemary
- ❖ 1 teaspoon salt
- ❖ ½ teaspoon black pepper
- ❖ 1 refrigerated pie crust, rolled out (optional)
- ❖ Fresh parsley, chopped (for garnish)

INSTRUCTIONS

1. Place chicken cubes in slow cooker.
2. Include Vegetables: Top chicken with onion, potatoes, corn, and carrots.
3. Include seasonings: Add chicken broth. Mix in salt, pepper, thyme, and minced garlic.
4. Cover and simmer the slow cooker on low for 6–8 hours or high for 3–4 hours to cook the chicken and vegetables.
5. Reduce Filling Thickness: Blend flour and heavy cream in a small bowl. In the last 30 minutes of simmering, stir this

mixture into the slow cooker. Cook until the filling thickens.

6. Bake pie crust if desired: Set your oven to 400°F (200°C) for a traditional pie crust. Roll out and bake the pie dough until golden brown per the package instructions. Break and place over chicken mixture when ready to serve.

7. Serve: Pour hot chicken pot pie into dishes, sprinkle with fresh parsley, and top with pie crust bits if preferred.

NOTE

➢ Crust Substitutes: Instead of making a separate pie crust, you can serve the chicken pot pie with puff pastry or biscuits.

➢ Variations with Vegetables: Feel free to include or omit other veggies such as celery, mushrooms, or green beans.

➢ Storage:

➢ Refrigerate leftovers for three days or freeze them for three months in an airtight container.

➢ Rewarm pot pie filling in a saucepan or microwave. For crispness, microwave the pie crust separately.

INGREDIENTS

For the Meatballs:

- ❖ 1 pound (450 g) ground beef or pork
- ❖ 1/4 cup grated Parmesan cheese
- ❖ 1/4 cup bread crumbs
- ❖ 1/4 cup milk
- ❖ 1 large egg
- ❖ 2 cloves garlic, minced
- ❖ 1 teaspoon dried Italian seasoning
- ❖ 1/2 teaspoon salt
- ❖ 1/4 teaspoon black pepper

For the Soup:

- ❖ 8 cups chicken broth
- ❖ 1 small onion, finely chopped
- ❖ 2 cloves garlic, minced
- ❖ 3 medium carrots, sliced
- ❖ 2 celery stalks, sliced
- ❖ Acini di pepe or other little pasta, 1 cup
- ❖ 4 cups fresh spinach or escarole, chopped
- ❖ Salt and pepper to taste
- ❖ Grated Parmesan cheese for serving
- ❖ Fresh parsley, chopped (for garnish)

INSTRUCTIONS

1. In a large bowl, combine ground pork or beef, bread crumbs, Parmesan cheese, milk, egg, minced garlic, Italian seasoning, salt, and pepper to make meatballs.
2. Form them into 1-inch meatballs. Put away.
3. Start the soup foundation by placing the meatballs in the slow cooker from the bottom up.
4. Mix minced garlic, diced onion, sliced carrots, and celery with chicken stock.
5. Make Soup:
6. Cover the slow cooker and stew on low for six to eight hours or high for 3–4 hours after cooking the meatballs with vegetables.
7. Put pasta and greens in.
8. In the last 30 minutes, add acini di pepe pasta and chopped escarole or spinach. Mix well to combine. Cook pasta till tender.
9. After tasting, add salt and pepper to the soup.
10. Top with grated Parmesan and chopped parsley and serve hot.

NOTE

➢ Mixing ground veal, pork, and beefmakes flavorful meatballs.
➢ Alternatives: Ditalini or orzo can replace acini di pepe.
➢ If you don't have spinach or escarole, try Swiss chard or kale.
➢ In an airtight container, leftovers can be frozen for three months or refrigerated for three days. As the pasta sits, some moisture may leak; reheat with more broth.

Reheat the soup in the microwave or on medium heat in a pot.

53. SLOW COOKER FRENCH ONION SOUP

INGREDIENTS

- ❖ 6 large onions, thinly sliced
- ❖ 3 tablespoons butter
- ❖ 2 tablespoons olive oil
- ❖ 1 tablespoon brown sugar
- ❖ 2 teaspoons salt
- ❖ 1 teaspoon black pepper
- ❖ 1 teaspoon dried thyme
- ❖ 1/2 cup dry white wine (optional)
- ❖ 8 cups beef broth
- ❖ 1 bay leaf
- ❖ 1 baguette, sliced
- ❖ 2 cups grated Gruyère cheese

INSTRUCTIONS

1. In a large skillet, caramelize onions with butter and olive oil over medium heat.
2. Combine brown sugar, salt, pepper, and sliced onions.
3. Stir occasionally while simmering the onions for 20–25 minutes until caramelized and golden brown.
4. Move to Slow Cooker: Put caramelized onions in the slow cooker.
5. Mix in bay leaf, beef broth, and dried thyme.
6. Add white wine if using.
7. Mix everything.
8. Cook the Soup: Cover the soup and cook on low for 6–8 hours or high for 3–4 hours until fragrant and flavorful.
9. Prepare cheese and bread:

10. Ten minutes before serving, broil on high in the oven.
11. Toast baguette slices on a baking sheet for one to two minutes per side until golden brown.
12. Ladle heated soup into
13. oven-safe bowls to serve.
14. Add toasted bread and grated Gruyère cheese to each bowl.
15. Place the bowls under the broiler for two to three minutes after the cheese melts and bubbles.
16. Serve immediately, with additional thyme if desired.

NOTE:

- Combine sweet and yellow onions for deeper flavor.
- Wine: You can remove the white wine, but it adds acidity.
- Gruyère can be replaced with Swiss cheese or a blend of mozzarella and parmesan.
- Store leftovers in an airtight container. It keeps for three days in the fridge. To avoid sogginess, they are stored separately.
- Reheating: Heat the soup in the microwave or pot over medium heat until warm. Toast fresh baguette slices and add cheese before serving.

INGREDIENTS

- ❖ 2 cups dried lentils (red or yellow), rinsed and drained
- ❖ 1 large onion, finely chopped
- ❖ 3 cloves garlic, minced
- ❖ 1 tablespoon fresh ginger, minced
- ❖ 1 can (14.5 oz) diced tomatoes
- ❖ 4 cups vegetable broth or water
- ❖ 1 can (14 oz) coconut milk
- ❖ 2 teaspoons ground cumin
- ❖ 2 teaspoons ground coriander
- ❖ 1 teaspoon turmeric
- ❖ 1 teaspoon garam masala
- ❖ 1 teaspoon salt (adjust to taste)
- ❖ 1/2 teaspoon cayenne pepper (optional for heat)
- ❖ 1 teaspoon mustard seeds
- ❖ 1 teaspoon cumin seeds
- ❖ 2 tablespoons olive oil or ghee
- ❖ Fresh cilantro, chopped (for garnish)
- ❖ Lemon wedges (for serving)

1. Get the ingredients ready by draining and rinsing the lentils.
2. Mince the ginger and garlic, then finely chop the onion.

Blend in Slow Cooker:

1. In the slow cooker, combine the lentils, diced tomatoes, onion, garlic, ginger, turmeric, garam masala, ground cumin, ground coriander, coconut milk, salt, and cayenne pepper (if using).
2. Mix everything.

Prepare Dal:

1. Cover the lentils and cook for 6-8 hours on low or 3-4 hours on high until mushy and flavorful.

Prepare Tadka (tempering):

1. On medium, heat ghee or olive oil in a small skillet.
2. Add the cumin and mustard seeds. Cook for one to two minutes or until they begin to pop and smell aromatic.
3. After adding the tadka to the slow cooker with the cooked dal, stir it quickly.

Serve the lentil dal hot, with lemon wedges on the side and fresh cilantro as a garnish.

NOTE:

- ➢ Alternative Lentils: While brown or green lentils take more time to cook, yellow or red lentils are better since they cook quickly and have a creamy texture.
- ➢ Consistency: If the dal is too thin, add extra water or vegetable broth to adjust its thickness. Otherwise, cook it uncovered for thirty minutes.
- ➢ Spice Level: Adjust the cayenne pepper to regulate the degree of heat. For added spiciness, add chopped green chile.
- ➢ Serving Ideas: For a full dinner, serve the dal with roti, rice, or naan.
- ➢ Refrigerate leftovers for 4 days or freeze for 3 months in an airtight container.
- ➢ If needed, add water or broth to the dal and reheat in the microwave or saucepan over medium heat.

55. SLOW COOKER BEEF AND BROCCOLI

INGREDIENTS

- ❖ 1 ½ pounds beef chuck or flank steak, thinly sliced
- ❖ 1 cup beef broth
- ❖ 1/2 cup soy sauce
- ❖ 1/4 cup brown sugar
- ❖ 2 tablespoons sesame oil
- ❖ 4 cloves garlic, minced
- ❖ 1 tablespoon fresh ginger, minced
- ❖ 1/4 cup oyster sauce
- ❖ 1/4 cup cornstarch
- ❖ 4 cups broccoli florets
- ❖ Cooked white rice or noodles (for serving)
- ❖ Sesame seeds (for garnish, optional)
- ❖ Sliced green onions (for garnish, optional)

INSTRUCTIONS

1. Thinly slice flank steak or beef chuck.
2. Finely chop ginger and garlic.
3. Add to slow cooker: Mix brown sugar, sesame oil, soy sauce, minced ginger and garlic, and beef broth in the slow cooker.
4. Mix the ingredients into the sliced steak to coat evenly.
5. Tenderize beef and simmer covered for 4-5 hours on low or 2-3 on high.
6. In a small dish, whisk together the cornstarch and 1/4 cup liquid to thicken the sauce in the slow cooker.
7. Return slurry and oyster sauce to slow cooker. Mix well.
8. Add broccoli florets to slow cooker.

9. Cook. After the broccoli is cooked and the sauce thickens, cover and cook on high for 30 minutes.

Serve:

- Top steak and broccoli with hot white rice or noodles.
- If desired, add chopped green onions and sesame seeds.

NOTE:

- ➤ Note that flank steak or beef chuck work well with this recipe. Finely slice beef to cook evenly.
- ➤ Choose fresh broccoli over frozen. Add frozen broccoli in the last 15 minutes.
- ➤ Increase cornstarch slurry to thicken sauce.
- ➤ Add rice vinegar or hoisin sauce for flavor.
- ➤ Airtight containers can keep leftovers in the fridge for three days. Freeze beef and broccoli for three months.
- ➤ Rewarm on medium in microwave or saucepan.

56. SLOW COOKER PEKING DUCK

INGREDIENTS

- ❖ 1 whole duck (about 4-5 pounds)
- ❖ 1/4 cup soy sauce
- ❖ 1/4 cup hoisin sauce
- ❖ 2 tablespoons honey
- ❖ 1 tablespoon Chinese five-spice powder
- ❖ 1 tablespoon fresh ginger, minced
- ❖ 4 cloves garlic, minced
- ❖ 1/3 cups dry sherry or rice wine
- ❖ 2 green onions, sliced
- ❖ 1 cucumber, julienned
- ❖ 12 Chinese pancakes or flour tortillas
- ❖ Hoisin sauce (for serving)

INSTRUCTIONS

Get the duck ready:

1. After washing the duck in cold water, blot dry it with paper towels.
2. Use a fork or skewer to make several holes in the skin to help render fat during cooking.

Prepare the marinade:

1. Mix the rice wine or dry sherry, soy sauce, hoisin sauce, honey, Chinese five-spice powder, minced ginger, and minced garlic in a bowl.

2. To marinate the duck, put it in a shallow dish or a sizable zip-top bag. After pouring the marinade over it, make sure the duck is evenly coated.
3. Refrigerate the dish or bag for at least four hours or overnight for best results.
4. To cook the duck, remove it from the marinade and set it in the slow cooker. Cover the duck with any leftover marinade.
5. Cook the duck for 6 to 8 hours on low, covered, or until the meat falls off the bone.
6. Preheat oven broiler toPreheat the oven broiler to crisp the skin, optional but recommended. The duck should be carefully removed from the slow cooker and placed on a baking tray.
7. To get golden, crispy skin, broiled the duck for 5–10 minutes. Watch to prevent fire.
8. Make pancakes: While the duck broils, reheat flour tortillas or Chinese pancakes according to package instructions.

Duck meat should be shred and skin removed before serving.

Serve duck with hoisin sauce, cucumber, green scallions, and hot pancakes. Put hoisin sauce on a pancake, add duck, cucumber, and green onions, then roll it up.

NOTE:

- ➤ Choose Your Duck: If a whole duck isn't available, you may substitute duck legs or breasts; modify the cooking timings.
- ➤ Marinating Time: Leave the duck in the marinade overnight for maximum flavor.
- ➤ Crisping the Skin: Although not required, crisping the skin under a broiler produces a more realistic texture and flavor.
- ➤ Serving suggestion: Although flour tortillas make a good stand-in for thin pancakes, they are traditionally served with Peking duck.
- ➤ Storage: KeepLeftovers can be stored in the fridge for up to three days in an airtight container. To keep the skin crispy, reheat in the oven.

INGREDIENTS

- ❖ 4 boneless, skinless chicken breasts
- ❖ 1 cup Italian seasoned bread crumbs
- ❖ 1/2 cup grated Parmesan cheese
- ❖ 1 teaspoon dried basil
- ❖ 1 teaspoon dried oregano
- ❖ 1/2 teaspoon garlic powder
- ❖ 1/2 teaspoon salt
- ❖ 1/2 teaspoon black pepper
- ❖ 1 large egg
- ❖ 1 cup marinara sauce
- ❖ 1 1/2 cups shredded mozzarella cheese
- ❖ 1/2 cup shredded Parmesan cheese
- ❖ Fresh basil or parsley, chopped (for garnish)
- ❖ Cooked pasta (for serving)

INSTRUCTIONS

1. To make the coating, combine the Parmesan cheese, dried oregano, dried basil, garlic powder, salt, and black pepper in a shallow bowl with the Italian-seasoned bread crumbs.
2. To wash the egg, beat the egg in a different shallow basin.
3. Coat the Chicken: Dredge each breast of chicken in the beaten egg, then wholly coat it in the bread crumbs mixture, pressing the crumbs firmly to stick to the chicken.
4. Slow cooker bottoms should have one layer of breaded chicken breasts.
5. Evenly coat chicken breasts with marinara.

6. Cook chicken: Low for 5–6 hours or high for 2–3 hours until tender and done.
7. Sprinkle grated Parmesan and mozzarella over chicken in the last 30 minutes. Cover and melt cheese.

Serve:

- Garnish the chicken with parsley or fresh basil and serve it hot.
- Serve with cooked pasta and, if preferred, additional marinara sauce on the side.

NOTE:

- ➤ Chicken Thickness: For more even cooking, pound or butterfly extremely thick chicken breasts to a uniform thickness.
- ➤ Cheese Options: You can use a mixture of provolone and mozzarella cheese for a deeper flavor.
- ➤ Sauce: Create your own marinara sauce, or use your favorite for a more flavorful version.
- ➤ Option for Crisping: After cooking, you can broil the chicken briefly if you'd like a crispier coating. After taking the chicken breasts out of the slow cooker, put them on a baking sheet and broil them for a few minutes to brown and bubble the cheese.
- ➤ Storage: Leftovers can be stored in an airtight container in the fridge for up to three days. They can then be reheated in a microwave or oven.

INGREDIENTS

- ❖ 1 ½ pounds fragmented boneless and skinless chicken thighs
- ❖ 1 large onion, chopped
- ❖ 3 cloves garlic, minced
- ❖ 1 tablespoon fresh ginger, minced
- ❖ 2 tablespoons red curry paste
- ❖ 1 can (14 oz) coconut milk
- ❖ 1 cup chicken broth
- ❖ 1 tablespoon soy sauce
- ❖ 1 tablespoon fish sauce
- ❖ 1 tablespoon brown sugar
- ❖ 2 cups diced tomatoes (fresh or canned)
- ❖ 2 cups baby spinach or kale, chopped
- ❖ 1 red bell pepper, sliced
- ❖ 1 yellow bell pepper, sliced
- ❖ 1 tablespoon lime juice
- ❖ Fresh cilantro, chopped (for garnish)
- ❖ Cooked rice or naan (for serving)

INSTRUCTIONS

1. Get the ingredients ready:
2. Tear the chicken thighs into large pieces.
3. Cut the onion and mince the garlic and ginger.
4. Slow-cooker blend:
5. Put chicken cubes in slow cooker.
6. Stir in red curry paste, garlic, ginger, and chopped onion. Stir curry paste into chicken.
7. Include Liquids:
8. Add the brown sugar, soy sauce, fish sauce, coconut milk, and chicken broth. Mix everything.
9. Add the diced tomatoes to the slow cooker.
10. Prepare the chicken:
11. Once the chicken is cooked through and tender, simmer it covered for 6–8 hours on low or 3–4 hours on high.
12. Add Vegetables: Sliced red and yellow bell peppers and baby spinach or kale should be added during the final 30 minutes of simmering. Mix everything.
13. Incorporate the lime juice and adjust the flavor by adding extra soy sauce, fish sauce, or brown sugar.

Serve:

- Warm coconut curry chicken with naan bread or overcooked rice.
- Add fresh cilantro as a garnish.

NOTE:

➤ Chicken Options: You can use skinless, boneless chicken breasts instead of the thighs.
➤ Variations with Vegetables: Feel free to add different veggies, such as peas, carrots, or green beans.
➤ Spice Level: To control the heat level, adjust the quantity of red curry paste. For added spiciness, you can also add a chopped chile.
➤ Use full-fat coconut milk for creamier curry. Use mild coconut milk.
➤ Refrigerate leftovers for three days or freeze them for three months in an airtight container.
➤ Reheat curry in microwave or saucepan on medium.

INGREDIENTS

- ❖ 2 pounds boneless lamb shoulder and cut into cubes
- ❖ 2 tablespoons olive oil
- ❖ 1 large onion, chopped
- ❖ 3 cloves garlic, minced
- ❖ 2 teaspoons ground cumin
- ❖ 2 teaspoons ground coriander
- ❖ 1 teaspoon ground cinnamon
- ❖ 1 teaspoon ground ginger
- ❖ 1/2 teaspoon ground turmeric
- ❖ 1/2 teaspoon ground paprika
- ❖ 1/4 teaspoon ground cloves
- ❖ 1/4 teaspoon ground nutmeg
- ❖ 1/4 teaspoon cayenne pepper (optional for heat)
- ❖ Salt and black pepper to taste
- ❖ 1 cup chicken or lamb broth
- ❖ 1 can (14 oz) diced tomatoes, undrained
- ❖ 1/2 cup dried apricots, chopped
- ❖ 1/2 cup raisins
- ❖ 1/4 cup chopped fresh cilantro
- ❖ 1/4 cup chopped fresh parsley
- ❖ Cooked couscous or rice (for serving)

INSTRUCTIONS

1. Place a large skillet over medium-high heat with olive oil to sear the lamb.
2. Black pepper and salt are used to season the lamb cubes.
3. In the skillet, sear the lamb cubes for about five minutes or until browned all over. Then, transfer the lamb to the slow cooker.
4. To prepare the aromatics, add minced garlic and diced onion to the same skillet. Cook for 3–4 minutes or until tender.
5. Include ground cloves, nutmeg, paprika, cumin, coriander, cinnamon, ginger, turmeric, and cayenne pepper (if using). Cook, stirring regularly, for another minute.
6. Add all ingredients to the slow cooker.
7. Stir onion and spices into slow cooker with seared lamb.
8. Add juices, sliced tomatoes, and chicken or lamb broth.
9. Add the raisins and chopped dry apricots.

Prepare the tagline:

1. Cook the lamb covered for 6-8 hours on low or 3-4 hours on high or until it is tender and the flavors are well combined.
2. To finish and serve, add the freshly chopped parsley and cilantro and stir.
3. Warm up the Moroccan Lamb Tagine and serve it over rice or prepared couscous.

NOTE:

- ➢ Lamb Shoulder: Slow cooking brings out the taste and tenderness of lamb shoulder.
- ➢ Spice Level: Modify the cayenne pepper quantity to your desired level of spiciness.
- ➢ Dried Fruit: Raisins and dried apricots give the meal a pleasant touch. For diversity, you can also use dates or prunes.
- ➢ Veggies: To add texture and taste, add veggies like potatoes, carrots, or bell peppers.
- ➢ Storage: Keep leftovers sealed. The fridge can hold them for three days. Reheat gently in the microwave or stove before serving.

INGREDIENTS

- ❖ 2 pounds of beef stew meat and cut into cubes
- ❖ 2 tablespoons vegetable oil
- ❖ 2 large onions, chopped
- ❖ 3 cloves garlic, minced
- ❖ 2 tablespoons paprika
- ❖ 1 teaspoon caraway seeds
- ❖ 1 teaspoon dried thyme
- ❖ 1 teaspoon dried marjoram
- ❖ 1 bay leaf
- ❖ Salt and black pepper to taste
- ❖ 1 can (14.5 oz) diced tomatoes, undrained
- ❖ 2 cups beef broth
- ❖ 2 large potatoes, peeled and diced
- ❖ 2 carrots, peeled and sliced
- ❖ 1 green bell pepper, diced
- ❖ 1 red bell pepper, diced
- ❖ 1/4 cup sour cream (optional for serving)
- ❖ Chopped fresh parsley (for garnish)
- ❖ Serving dish: cooked egg noodles or crusty toast

1. Sear meat in vegetable oil in a large skillet over medium-high heat.
2. Add black pepper and salt to the meat cubes.
3. Sear beef cubes for five minutes in the skillet until browned. On the low heat stove, place the steak.
4. Sautée Aromatiques: Add chopped onions and minced garlic to the skillet. Cook until tender, 3–4 minutes.
5. Add dried thyme, marjoram, caraway, paprika, and bay leaf. Continuously stir and fry another minute.

Mix items in slow cooker:

1. Put seared meat, onion, and spices in the slow cooker.
2. Put beef broth and diced tomatoes with
3. liquids in the slow cooker.
4. Cover and simmer goulash for 6–8 hours on low or 3–4 hours on high until beef is very tender.
5. During the last hour of cooking, add sliced carrots, diced red bell pepper, chopped green bell pepper, and diced potatoes to the slow cooker. Mix well to combine.
6. Finally, remove the bay leaf and serve.
7. Serve hot Hungarian goulash with fresh parsley.
8. To thicken, add sour cream before serving.
9. Serve with cooked egg noodles or crusty bread.

NOTE:

➢ Use chuck roast or beef stew for best results. Remove excess fat before cooking.

➢ For real flavor, try Hungarian sweet paprika, but normal paprika will work too.

➢ Hungarian goulash tastes peculiar with caraway seeds. If they're unavailable, add cumin seeds or leave them out.

➢ Add celery, mushrooms, or tomatoes for variety.

➢ Keep leftovers refrigerated in an airtight container. Before serving, reheat gently in the microwave or on the stovetop.

61. SLOW COOKER CHICKEN AND RICE

INGREDIENTS

- ❖ 1 and a half pounds of boneless, skinless chicken breasts or thighs and cut into small pieces
- ❖ Drain and rinse one and a half cups long-grain white rice.
- ❖ 1 onion, chopped
- ❖ 3 cloves garlic, minced
- ❖ 1 red bell pepper, chopped
- ❖ 1 green bell pepper, chopped
- ❖ 1 can (14.5 oz) diced tomatoes, undrained
- ❖ 2 cups chicken broth
- ❖ 1 teaspoon dried thyme
- ❖ 1 teaspoon dried oregano
- ❖ 1 teaspoon paprika
- ❖ Salt and black pepper to taste
- ❖ Fresh parsley, chopped (for garnish)

INSTRUCTIONS

1. Combine Ingredients in Slow Cooker: Fill the slow cooker with the diced tomatoes (with their liquids), chopped onion, minced garlic, chopped bell peppers, rinsed rice, and chicken broth.
2. Stir in the paprika, dried oregano, dry thyme, salt, and black pepper. Mix everything.
3. Get the chicken
4. and rice cooked.
5. Let cook for 6-8 hours on low or *3-4 hours on high until rice is mushy and chicken is done.*
6. *Fork-fluff the chicken and rice before serving.*

7. *Add some fresh parsley before serving.*

NOTE:

- ➤ Options for Chicken: You can use skinless, boneless chicken thighs or breasts, depending on your taste.
- ➤ Rice: To avoid clumping, rinse the rice before putting it in the slow cooker.
- ➤ Vegetables: For more taste and nutrition, add additional vegetables like spinach, carrots, or peas.
- ➤ Broth: You may use store-bought or homemade chicken broth. If using store-bought broth, adjust the salt proportionately.
- ➤ Spices: Tailor the spice mixture to your preference. You can add smoked paprika, chili powder, or cumin for more flavor.
- ➤ Storage: In an airtight container, keep leftovers in the fridge for up to three days. If necessary, reheat slowly in the microwave or stovetop and moisten with a splash of broth or water.

62. SLOW COOKER POTATO LEEK SOUP

INGREDIENTS

- ❖ 4 cups of vegetable or chicken broth
- ❖ 1 cup of milk or cream
- ❖ 2 minced garlic cloves
- ❖ 4 medium potatoes (peeled and diced
- ❖) 4 large leeks (white and light green parts only)
- ❖ 2 tablespoons butter
- ❖ Salt and black pepper to taste
- ❖ Chopped fresh chives or parsley (for garnish)

INSTRUCTIONS

1. Before you start to assemble the ingredients, make sure the sliced leeks are clean by rinsing them under cold water.
2. Clean and slice the potatoes.
3. Go ahead and put everything in the slow cooker.
4. In a slow cooker, combine the diced potatoes, chopped garlic, sliced leeks, and broth (chicken or vegetarian option is available).
5. Salt and black pepper can be added according to taste.
6. Slow boil the butter in a saucepan.
7. Make the Soup: Simmer, covered, for 6–8 hours on low heat or 3–4 hours on moderate heat, or until potatoes are tender.
8. Get the Soup Blended: Make sure the soup is completely smooth and creamy by blending it with an immersion blender. However, you could blend the soup in batches. Hot soup requires caution.

9. Milk or cream can be added to blended soup to make it creamier. Adjust the quantity to your desire.
10. Season soup with salt and pepper.
11. Serve hot potato leek soup on each platter.
12. Sprinkle fresh chives or chopped parsley for presentation.

NOTE:

➢ Creaminess: Milk or cream might enhance this soup's flavor, but it's not required. Try coconut milk or another dairy-free option for plant-based eating.

➢ Options: Add white wine or chopped fresh herbs like thyme or rosemary after cooking to enhance the flavor.

➢ Refrigeration: Remaining food can be kept fresh for four days in airtight containers. Return it to the oven or microwave for a final warm before serving.

➢ This soup freezes well. Cool thoroughly and transfer to freezer-safe containers. Freeze it for three months. Thaw overnight in the fridge before heating.

➢ Texture: Blend half the ingredients and leave some potato and leek bits for a chunkier soup.

63. SLOW COOKER EGGPLANT PARMESAN

INGREDIENTS

- ❖ 2 large eggplants, sliced into 1/2-inch rounds
- ❖ Salt
- ❖ 2 cups breadcrumbs (Italian seasoned breadcrumbs work well)
- ❖ 1 cup grated Parmesan cheese
- ❖ 2 eggs, beaten
- ❖ 2 cups marinara sauce
- ❖ 2 cups shredded mozzarella cheese
- ❖ Fresh basil leaves, chopped (for garnish)
- ❖ Cooked spaghetti or crusty bread (for serving)

INSTRUCTIONS

1. To start, slice the eggplant and place it in a strainer. Sprinkle with salt and pepper to taste. Allow them to drain for around thirty minutes in order to remove any excess moisture. Doing so will keep the eggplant from becoming overcooked.
2. To coat the eggplant, soak the slices in cold water for 30 minutes, then pat them dry with paper towels.
3. In a small bowl, mix together the breadcrumbs and grated Parmesan cheese.
4. Press each eggplant slice lightly to adhere after dipping into the beaten eggs and covering with the breadcrumb mixture.
5. Begin by lightly coating the bottom of the slow cooker with marinara sauce.
6. Breaded eggplant

7. slices should be layered on top of the sauce.
8. In a baking dish, arrange sliced eggplant, marinara sauce, and shredded mozzarella cheese in descending order of use. The finishing touch is a layer of marinara sauce and mozzarella cheese.

Cook:

- Cover and cook for 4–5 hours on low or 2–3 hours on high, or until the eggplant is soft and the cheese is bubbling and melted.

Present:

- Present the hot eggplant parmesan dish adorned with finely chopped, fresh basil leaves.
- Savor with prepared spaghetti or a side of crusty toast.

NOTE

- ➢ When slicing eggplant, try to get consistent slices for even cooking.
- ➢ Breading: For a lighter version, omit the breading step and arrange the cheese and sauce layers on the eggplant slices.
- ➢ Variations: To add more flavor and texture, you can sandwich sliced fresh tomatoes or ricotta cheese between the layers.
- ➢ Storage: In an airtight container, keep leftovers in the fridge for up to three days. Before serving, gently reheat in the oven or microwave.
- ➢ Eggplant Parmesan freezes quite nicely. Divide it and store it in freezer-safe containers for up to three months after cooling. Let it thaw overnight in the fridge before heating.

64. SLOW COOKER CUBAN BLACK BEANS

INGREDIENTS

- ❖ 1 pound dried black beans and rinsed, soaked overnight
- ❖ 1 large onion, chopped
- ❖ 1 green bell pepper, chopped
- ❖ 1 red bell pepper, chopped
- ❖ 4 cloves garlic, minced
- ❖ 2 bay leaves
- ❖ 1 teaspoon ground cumin
- ❖ 1 teaspoon dried oregano
- ❖ 1 teaspoon smoked paprika
- ❖ 1 teaspoon ground coriander
- ❖ 1/2 teaspoon cayenne pepper (adjust to taste)
- ❖ 4 cups vegetable or chicken broth
- ❖ 2 tablespoons tomato paste
- ❖ 2 tablespoons white vinegar
- ❖ Salt and black pepper to taste
- ❖ Fresh cilantro, chopped (for garnish)
- ❖ Cooked white rice (for serving)

INSTRUCTIONS

1. Prepare the ingredients by rinsing and soaking the dried black beans in water for the entire night. Before using, drain.
2. Mix the red and green bell peppers with the onion and chop them. Garlic, diced.
3. Put everything into the slow cooker at this time.
4. Soak the black beans, then add the chopped onion, bell peppers, minced garlic, bay leaves, ground cumin, dried

oregano, ground coriander, smoked paprika, and cayenne pepper to the slow cooker.

5. Pour the vegetable or chicken broth after adding the tomato paste and white vinegar. Mix everything together.

Prepare the Beans:

1. Once black beans are soft, cover and simmer on low for 8–10 hours or high for 4–6.
2. Remove bay leaves and season beans to tasteafter cooking.
3. Add salt and black pepper to taste.
4. Boil white rice and serve Cuban black beans warm.
5. Chop cilantro and garnish.

NOTE:

➢ Black beans: Black beans that have been soaked overnight have a better texture and require less boiling time.
➢ Vegetables: Feel free to change the quantity of onions and bell peppers to suit your tastes.
➢ Spices: To control the degree of spiciness, adjust the amount of cayenne pepper. For added spice, you can also add a diced jalapeño pepper.
➢ Tomato Paste: Tomato paste gives the beans a richer flavor.
➢ Storage:An airtight container can keep leftovers in the fridge for four days. Reheat gently in the microwave or stove before serving.
➢ Cuban black beans freeze well. After cooling, separate them and store in freezer-safe containers for three months. Let it thaw overnight in the fridge before heating.

INGREDIENTS

- ❖ 2 pounds bone-in, skin-on chicken thighs (you can use boneless, skinless if preferred)
- ❖ 1/2 cup soy sauce
- ❖ 1/4 cup white vinegar
- ❖ 1/4 cup apple cider vinegar
- ❖ 1/4 cup water
- ❖ 4 cloves garlic, minced
- ❖ 1 onion, sliced
- ❖ 3 bay leaves
- ❖ 1 teaspoon whole black peppercorns
- ❖ 1 teaspoon brown sugar (optional)
- ❖ Cooked rice (for serving)
- ❖ Chopped green onions or cilantro (for garnish)

INSTRUCTIONS

1. Cook the Chicken: Remove or keep the skin on skin-on, bone-in chicken thighs. Trim excess fat.
2. Put everything in the slow cooker.
3. In the slow cooker
4. , add soy sauce, white vinegar, apple cider vinegar, water, sliced onion, minced garlic, bay leaves, whole black peppercorns, and brown sugar (if using). Mix everything.
5. Put chicken in slow cooker:
6. In the slow cooker, cover chicken thighs with marinade.
7. Make Adobo Chicken:
8. Simmer covered for 6–8 hours on low or 3–4 hours on highafter the chicken is tender.

9. Remove Chicken Adobo from the slow cooker and place on a platter.
10. You can filter
11. or remove fat from the sauce.
12. Serve hot adobo chicken over rice with sauce.
13. Add chopped cilantro or green onions for flavor and color.

NOTE:

- ➢ Chicken thighs: Skinless, boneless chicken thighs can be used to make chicken adobo.
- ➢ For better flavor, marinate the chicken in the sauce for several hours or overnight.
- ➢ Coconut milk, pineapple juice, bay leaves, and whole peppercorns make chicken adobo.
- ➢ Traditionally eaten over rice, chicken adobo can be served with toast, potatoes, or noodles.
- ➢ Refrigerate leftovers for three days in an airtight container. Reheat gently in the microwave or stove before serving.

INGREDIENTS

- ❖ 2 pounds beef chuck roast, cut into large chunks
- ❖ 1 onion, chopped
- ❖ 3 cloves garlic, minced
- ❖ 1 can (14.5 oz) diced tomatoes, undrained
- ❖ 2 tablespoons tomato paste
- ❖ 1 tablespoon chili powder
- ❖ 1 teaspoon ground cumin
- ❖ 1 teaspoon smoked paprika
- ❖ 1 teaspoon dried oregano
- ❖ 1/2 teaspoon ground coriander
- ❖ Salt and black pepper to taste
- ❖ 1/2 cup beef broth
- ❖ Corn or flour tortillas (for serving)
- ❖ Optional toppings: shredded lettuce, diced tomatoes, shredded cheese, sliced jalapeños, chopped cilantro, sour cream, guacamole, salsa

INSTRUCTIONS

1. Mince garlic and cut onion.
2. Break roast beef chuck into pieces.
3. Put everything into the slow cooker and stir.
4. Put everything into the slow cooker: diced tomatoes with juices, minced onion, chopped garlic, chopped onion, tomato paste, smoked paprika, ground cumin, ground coriander, dried oregano, ground coriander, salt, and black pepper. Combine the meat pieces and mix thoroughly.
5. After adding the beef broth, combine all the ingredients.
6. Bring the beef to a simmer in a saucepan. When cooked for 8 hours on low heat or 4 hours on high heat, covered and simmering, the beef should be tender enough to shred with a fork.
7. Separating the meat: Shred the cooked beef with two forks in the slow cooker, then mix it with the sauce.
8. Prior to eating, reheat the tortillas according to the package's instructions.
9. Warm the tortillas and spread a little of the shredded beef mixture on top.
10. Garnish with salsa, guacamole, sour cream, cilantro, shredded cheese, sliced tomatoes, lettuce, and whichever salsa you like most.

NOTE:

- ➢ Chuck roast meat becomes juicy and delicious when cooked slowly. Additionally, we have beef brisket and beef shoulder.
- ➢ Toss on some toppings of your choice to make your tacos uniquely yours. Some of the most typical combinations are cheese, cabbage, tomatoes, jalapeños, sour cream, avocado, and salsa.
- ➢ You may store any leftover beef for up to three days in the fridge if you seal it in a container. A quick warming in the microwave or on low heat just before serving will do the trick.
- ➢ Beef filling freezes beautifully. After it has cooled entirely, put it in a jar that may be frozen for up to three months. Allow it to defrost in the fridge for at least one night prior to cooking.
- ➢ Personalization: The beef's flavor can be adjusted to your liking. Verify the flavor with a taste test and tweak the chili powder proportions as needed.

INGREDIENTS

- ❖ 2 pounds pork shoulder or pork loin and cut into cubes
- ❖ 2 tablespoons olive oil
- ❖ 1 onion, chopped
- ❖ 2 cloves garlic, minced
- ❖ 2 carrots, peeled and diced
- ❖ 2 celery stalks, diced
- ❖ 2 apples, peeled, cored, and diced
- ❖ 2 cups chicken broth
- ❖ 1 cup apple cider
- ❖ 2 tablespoons Dijon mustard
- ❖ 2 tablespoons maple syrup or honey
- ❖ 2 bay leaves
- ❖ 1 teaspoon dried thyme
- ❖ Salt and black pepper to taste
- ❖ 2 tablespoons cornstarch (optional for thickening)
- ❖ Chopped fresh parsley or thyme (for garnish)

INSTRUCTIONS

1. Place a large skillet over medium-high heat with olive oil to sear the pork.
2. Use salt and black pepper to season the pork cubes.
3. In the skillet, sear the pork cubes for about five minutes or until browned all over. Place the pork in the cooker set on low heat.
4. Saute Aromatics: In the same pan, add the chopped onion, celery, carrots, and garlic. Simmer until soft, about 5 minutes.

5. Add all ingredients to the slow cooker.
6. Add the seared pork and the sautéed vegetables to the slow cooker.
7. Add leaves, dried thyme, apple cider, Dijon mustard, maple syrup, honey, and chicken broth to the slow cooker. Mix ev to the slow cook everything.
8. Simmer the Stew: Cover and simmer on low for 6–8 hours or on high for 3–4 hours until the pork is cooked.
9. Optional: To thicken the stew, stir together 2 teaspoons of cornstarch and two tablespoons of cold water into a slurry. In the last half hour of cooking, stir the slurry into the stew. Simmer the stew until it thickens.

Serve:

- Remove the bay leaves from the stew after it has cooked.
- Garnish the Pork and Apple Stew with freshly chopped parsley or thyme and serve hot.

NOTE:

- ➢ Pork: Both loin and shoulder cuts of pork work well in this stew. Both cuts are top-notch, but the pork shoulder adds more flavor and tenderness to the stew due to its higher fat content.
- ➢ Apples: For this stew, choose for Braeburn or Granny Smith apples, which are firm and somewhat tart. They keep their form well when cooked and add a pleasant balance of acidity and sweetness.
- ➢ To thicken the stew, add a cornstarch slurry during the last 30 minutes of boiling. Another option is to cook the stew uncovered for a bit longer to reduce the sauce and thicken it.
- ➢ Preserving: If you make extra stew, cover it tightly and keep it in the fridge for three days. Warm it up little in the oven or microwave before serving.
- ➢ Freezing this stew is a breeze. Once cooled, transfer to airtight containers or freezer bags and keep for up to three months. Thaw overnight in the fridge
- ➢ before heating.

68. SLOW COOKER SPICED LENTILS

INGREDIENTS

- ❖ 2 cups dried lentils, rinsed and drained
- ❖ 1 onion, chopped
- ❖ 2 cloves garlic, minced
- ❖ 1 tablespoon ginger, minced
- ❖ 1 can (14.5 oz) diced tomatoes, undrained
- ❖ 3 cups vegetable broth
- ❖ 1 teaspoon ground cumin
- ❖ 1 teaspoon ground coriander
- ❖ 1/2 teaspoon ground turmeric
- ❖ 1/2 teaspoon ground cinnamon
- ❖ 1/4 teaspoon cayenne pepper (adjust to taste)
- ❖ Salt and black pepper to taste
- ❖ 1 cup coconut milk
- ❖ Fresh cilantro, chopped (for garnish)
- ❖ Cooked rice or naan bread (for serving)

INSTRUCTIONS

1. Ingredients to Combine: Rinse the lentils and add them to the slow cooker along with the diced tomatoes (with their juices), chopped onion, minced garlic, minced ginger, ground cumin, ground coriander, ground turmeric, ground cinnamon, cayenne pepper, salt, and black pepper. Mix everything.
2. Prepare the Lentils:
3. Cook the lentils covered for 6-8 hours on low or 3-4 hours on high or until they are soft and the flavors have combined.

4. Add Coconut Milk: In the final half-hour of cooking, stir in the coconut milk. This gives the lentils a creamier texture.
5. Taste the lentils and add salt, pepper, or spices if necessary to adjust the seasoning.

Serve:

➢ Top the hot spiced lentils with freshly chopped cilantro.
➢ Savor it with naan bread or boiled rice on the side.

NOTE:

➢ Lentils of any color will work in this recipe. Compared to brown or green lentils, which keep their shape better, red lentils are more likely to break down and have a creamier texture.
➢ Vegetables: Feel free to increase the nutritional value and flavor by adding extra vegetables, such as carrots, spinach, or bell peppers.
➢ Seasonings: Change the seasoning to your liking. Adjust cayenne pepper to your desired heat.
➢ Using full-fat coconut milk gives the lentils a rich, creamy flavor. Using light coconut milk will make it lighter.
➢ Safekeeping: MaintainYou can store any leftovers in the fridge for up to four days if they are sealed. Warm it up little in the oven or microwave before serving.
➢ Spiced lentils freeze well. After cooling, divide into parts and store in airtight containers to freeze for three months. Thaw overnight in the fridge before heating.

INGREDIENTS

- ❖ 2 pounds beef chuck roast and cut into 1-inch cubes
- ❖ 2 tablespoons vegetable oil
- ❖ 2 onions, chopped
- ❖ 3 cloves garlic, minced
- ❖ 2 tablespoons Hungarian sweet paprika
- ❖ 1 tablespoon tomato paste
- ❖ 1 teaspoon caraway seeds
- ❖ 1 teaspoon dried thyme
- ❖ 1 teaspoon dried marjoram
- ❖ 1 bay leaf
- ❖ Salt and black pepper to taste
- ❖ 2 cups beef broth
- ❖ 1 cup diced tomatoes (canned or fresh)
- ❖ 2 large potatoes, peeled and diced
- ❖ 2 carrots, peeled and sliced
- ❖ 1 green bell pepper, diced
- ❖ 1 red bell pepper, diced
- ❖ Chopped fresh parsley
- ❖ Cooked egg noodles or crusty bread

INSTRUCTION:

1. To brown the beef, heat the vegetable oil in a big skillet over medium-high heat.
2. Toss the beef pieces with some salt and black pepper.
3. To ensure even browning on both sides, fry the beef cubes in batches. Brown the steak and then transfer it to the slow cooker.

4. Seasoned Herbs: Toss in the chopped onions and minced garlic to the same pan. Simmer until soft, about 5 minutes.
5. To the tomato paste, add the caraway seeds, dried thyme, marjoram, bay leaf, and Hungarian sweet paprika. For an additional minute, cook while stirring often.
6. Go ahead and put everything in the slow cooker.
7. Once the beef has browned, place it in the slow cooker along with the onion and spice mixture.
8. Put the beef broth and diced tomatoes in the slow cooker. Blend all of the ingredients.
9. Simmer the goulash for 8–10 hours on low heat or 4–6 hours on high heat, or until the beef is tender. Cover and simmer.
10. In the last hourof cooking, add the veggies to the slow cooker: diced potatoes, sliced carrots, red and green bell peppers, and diced potatoes. Blend all of the ingredients.
11. Finalize and Present: Once the veggies have softened and the goulash has cooked, remove the bay leaf.
12. Add some freshly cut parsley on the *top of the hot Hungarian goulash before serving.*

Enjoy with a side of cooked egg noodles or crunchy bread.

NOTE:

- ➤ When cooked, chuck roast beef becomes soft and incredibly flavorful. Additional choices include beef round roast and stew meat.
- ➤ Paprika: Hungarian sweet paprika is the traditional ingredient in Hungarian goulash, but regular sweet paprika will do in a hurry.
- ➤ Add additional veggies, such as mushrooms, peas, or celery, for more flavor and texture.
- ➤ Preserving Food: Refrigerate leftovers for up to three days if sealed in a container. Warm it up little in the oven or microwave before serving.
- ➤ Freezing Hungarian goulash makes it taste even better. After it has cooled entirely, divide it into servings and store each one in a freezer-safe container; they will keep for up to three months. Before cooking, let it defrost in the fridge for at least one night.

INGREDIENTS

- ❖ 2 cups long-grain white rice
- ❖ 1 onion, finely chopped
- ❖ 1 bell pepper (red, green, or yellow), diced
- ❖ 2 cloves garlic, minced
- ❖ 1 can (14.5 oz) diced tomatoes, undrained
- ❖ 1 can (8 oz) tomato sauce
- ❖ 2 cups chicken broth or vegetable broth
- ❖ 1 teaspoon ground cumin
- ❖ 1 teaspoon chili powder
- ❖ 1/2 teaspoon paprika
- ❖ Salt and black pepper to taste
- ❖ Optional toppings: chopped fresh cilantro, diced avocado, sour cream, shredded cheese, lime wedges

INSTRUCTIONS

1. Instructions for Making a Slow Cooker Meal: Get everything ready by throwing everything into a slow cooker: A recipe that calls for long-grain white rice, diced tomatoes (including juice), diced bell pepper, chopped onion, minced garlic, tomato sauce, broth (either chicken or vegetable), ground cumin, paprika, chili powder, salt, and black pepper.

The rice should be rolled out:

1. Once the rice is cooked and most of the liquid has been absorbed, cover and simmer for two to three hours on low

heat (or one to two hours on high). Stir occasionally while cooking, especially in the last hour, to avoid sticking.

2. If you want the rice grains to show after cooking, fluff it with a fork. Following that, you should serve.

3. To serve, heat a serving dish and spoon the Spanish rice over top. If desired, top with avocado slices, sour cream, cilantro, lime wedges, or shredded cheese.

NOTE:

- ➢ This recipe calls for white long-grain rice, but brown or medium-grain rice would work just fine. Just change the amount of time it cooks for and the amount of liquid you use.
- ➢ The amount of chopped co
- ➢ rn, peas, or tomatoes you use can be adjusted to suit your desire in terms of flavor and texture of the vegetables.
- ➢ Seasonings: Tailor the blend of seasonings to your personal preference. The amount of chili powder and other spicescan be customized to suit individual taste.
- ➢ Avocado, sour cream, cheese, chopped cilantro, and lime wedges are a flavor explosion waiting to happen atop the Spanish rice.
- ➢ If you seal your leftover Spanish rice well, it will keep for three days in the fridge. Just give it a quick reheat in the oven or microwave before you serve it.
- ➢ The flavor of frozen Spanish rice is unparalleled. After it has cooled entirely, divide it into servings and store each one in a freezer-safe container; they will keep for up to three months. Put it in the fridge to thaw overnight before you cook it.

INGREDIENTS

- ❖ 1 pound chicken thighs, skinless and boneless, diced into bite-sized segments
- ❖ 1 onion, chopped
- ❖ 1 green bell pepper, chopped
- ❖ 2 celery stalks, chopped
- ❖ 3 cloves garlic, minced
- ❖ 1 can (14.5 oz) diced tomatoes, undrained
- ❖ 4 cups chicken broth
- ❖ 1/2 pound andouille sausage, sliced
- ❖ 1 cup okra, sliced (fresh or frozen)
- ❖ 2 bay leaves
- ❖ 1 teaspoon dried thyme
- ❖ 1 teaspoon dried oregano
- ❖ 1/2 teaspoon smoked paprika
- ❖ 1/4 teaspoon cayenne pepper (adjust to taste)
- ❖ Salt and black pepper to taste
- ❖ 1/4 cup all-purpose flour
- ❖ 1/4 cup vegetable oil
- ❖ Cooked white rice (for serving)
- ❖ Chopped fresh parsley or green onions

INSTRUCTIONS

1. Prepare the ingredients by chopping the chicken thighs into small pieces.
2. Finely chop the celery, green bell pepper, and onion.
3. Cut the andouille sausage into pieces.
4. Cut the okra into slices.

In the slow cooker, combine ingredients:

1. Add the diced tomatoes (with their juices), chopped celery, chopped onion, chopped green bell pepper, chopped smoked paprika, dried thyme, dried oregano, chopped okra, bay leaves, dried thyme, dried oregano, and cayenne pepper, salt, black pepper to the slow cooker. Mix well to blend.

Make the gumbo:

1. Once the chicken is thoroughly cooked and the flavors have been combined, and cover, cook on low for 6–8 hours or(on high for 3–4 hours).
2. Make Roux: Start the roux thirty minutes or so before the gumbo is finished cooking. Heat the vegetable oil over medium Pre-heat in a medium saucepan. Stir in the all-purpose flour gradually until smooth. Simmer the roux for approximately 15 to 20 minutes, stirring continuously, or until it turns a deep brown color.

Thicken Gumbo:

1. Slowly whisk the prepared roux into the gumbo in the slow cooker. Cook, stirring periodically, on high for a half hour or until the gumbo thickens.

Place the hot Chicken Gumbo on top of cooked white rice to serve.

Add green onions or finely chopped fresh parsley as a garnish.

NOTES:

- ➢ Prepare this dish using skinless, boneless poultry thighs or breasts. The flavor and moist consistency of quadriceps contribute to it's popularity.
- ➢ Andouille Sausage: The gumbo gains excellent flavor from the Andouille sausage. If it is unavailable, another spicy sausage can be used in its place.
- ➢ Okra: A traditional gumbo ingredient, okra lends a naturally thick consistency to the stew. If you dislike okra, leave it out, although the gumbo can have a slightly different texture.
- ➢ The roux is a necessary ingredient that gives the gumbo its thick consistency and rich, complex flavor. Make the roux slowly, ensuring it doesn't burn until it turns dark brown.
- ➢ Storage: You may keep any leftover chicken gumbo in an airtight container in the refrigerator for up to three days. Before serving, reheat gently over the stove or in the microwave.
- ➢ Gumbo freezes beautifully. Cool it completely, then freeze in freezer-safe containers for up to three months. Thaw overnight in the fridge before reheating.

72. SLOW COOKER PORK AND BEANS

INGREDIENTS

- ❖ 1 pound pork shoulder or pork loin, cut into chunks
- ❖ Two 15-ounce navy bean cans, drained and rinsed
- ❖ 1 onion, chopped
- ❖ 2 cloves garlic, minced
- ❖ 1/2 cup barbecue sauce
- ❖ 1/4 cup ketchup
- ❖ 2 tablespoons brown sugar
- ❖ 1 tablespoon mustard
- ❖ 1 tablespoon Worcestershire sauce
- ❖ Salt and black pepper to taste
- ❖ Optional toppings: chopped green onions, diced jalapeños, shredded cheese

INSTRUCTIONS

1. Prepare the ingredients by chopping the pork loin or shoulder into bite-sized pieces.
2. Recycle and empty the navy beans.
3. In the slow cooker, combine ingredients:
4. Add the chopped onion, minced garlic, drained navy beans, brown sugar, mustard, Worcestershire sauce, barbecue sauce, ketchup, salt, and black pepper to the pork chunks in the slow cooker. Mix well to blend.
5. Prepare the beans and pork:
6. After the pork is soft and the flavors have been combined, cover and simmer on low for 6–8 hours or on high for 3–4 hours.

To serve, taste after cooking and adjust the seasoning if necessary.

You can top the sizzling pork and beans with optional toppings like shredded cheese, diced jalapeños, or chopped green onions.

NOTE:

- ➢ Pork: This dish works well with pork shoulder or loin, with or without bones.
- ➢ Navy beans are a terrific option for this recipe, but you may also use pinto or Great Northern beans.
- ➢ To enhance the taste of the pork and beans, use your preferred barbecue sauce. Either homemade or store-bought barbecue sauce will work.
- ➢ Customization: Feel free to alter the recipe to suit your tastes and flavors. To add more sweetness, add more barbecue sauce; to add more tanginess, change the quantity of Worcestershire sauce and mustard.
- ➢ Storage: In an airtight container, keep leftovers in the fridge for up to three days. Before serving, reheat gently over the stove or in the microwave.
- ➢ Pork and beans make good freezer meals. Let cool thoroughly, then portion out and freeze in freezer-safe containers for up to 3 months. Thaw in the fridge for a whole night before reheating.

INGREDIENTS

- ❖ 1 pound boneless, skinless chicken breasts, diced
- ❖ 1 tablespoon olive oil
- ❖ 1 onion, finely chopped
- ❖ 2 carrots, diced
- ❖ 2 celery stalks, diced
- ❖ 3 cloves garlic, minced
- ❖ 1 tablespoon curry powder
- ❖ 1 teaspoon ground cumin
- ❖ One teaspoon of ground coriander
- ❖ 1/2 teaspoon ground turmeric
- ❖ 1/4 teaspoon cayenne pepper (adjust to taste)
- ❖ One can (14.5 oz) diced tomatoes, undrained
- ❖ 6 cups chicken broth
- ❖ 1 cup red lentils, rinsed
- ❖ 1/2 cup coconut milk
- ❖ Salt and black pepper to taste
- ❖ Fresh cilantro, chopped (for garnish)
- ❖ Cooked rice (for serving)

INSTRUCTIONS

1. Sauté aromatics in olive oil over medium heat. Add chopped carrots, celery, and onion. Cook until softened after 5 minutes. Use curry powder, cayenne pepper, ground cumin, coriander, turmeric, and sliced garlic. Stir often for 1–2 minutes until fragrant.
2. Mix everything
3. in a slow cooker. Mix in the spices and sautéed onion.

4. In a slow cooker, combine washed red lentils, diced chicken breasts, chicken broth, chopped tomatoes, and juices. Mix well to combine.
5. Tenderize the lentils and chicken before cooking the soup covered for 6-8 hours on low or 3-4 hours on high.
6. Add coconut milk *in the last 30 minutes.*

Sprinkle salt and pepper over soup before serving. Taste it after simmering.

Stir finely chopped fresh cilantro into heated Chicken Mulligatawny Soup.Reserve cooked rice.

NOTES:

- ➢ Chicken thighs can replace skinless, boneless breasts in the recipe.
- ➢ Red lentils are usually boiled briefly before adding to Mulligatawny soup. Rib them before slow cooking.
- ➢ That curry powder combo you love. Adjust the amount to taste and curry powder heat.
- ➢ Coconut milk decreases heat and thickens soup. Choose mild or full-fat coconut milk.
- ➢ Sprinkle chopped fresh cilantro on the soup for heat. Add yogurt or lime juice for extra flavor.
- ➢ Refrigerate leftovers in an airtight jar for three days. Microwave or low-heat.
- ➢ Freezing m
- ➢ ulligatawny soup is great. This can be frozen for three months after cooling. Heat after one hour of refrigeration.

74. SLOW COOKER PASTA E FAGIOLI

INGREDIENTS

- ❖ 1 tablespoon olive oil
- ❖ 1 onion, diced
- ❖ 2 carrots, diced
- ❖ 2 celery stalks, diced
- ❖ 3 cloves garlic, minced
- ❖ 1 can (14.5 oz) diced tomatoes, undrained
- ❖ One 15-ounce can of rinsed and drained red kidney beans
- ❖ Thirteen ounces of cannellini beans that have been rinsed and drained
- ❖ 4 cups vegetable broth or chicken broth
- ❖ 1 teaspoon dried oregano
- ❖ 1 teaspoon dried basil
- ❖ 1/2 teaspoon dried thyme
- ❖ 1/2 teaspoon dried rosemary
- ❖ 1/4 teaspoon red pepper flakes (optional)
- ❖ Salt ,black pepper to taste
- ❖ 1 cup small pasta
- ❖ Fresh parsley, chopped (for garnish)
- ❖ Grated Parmesan cheese (for serving)

Saute Aromatics:

1. In a skillet, gently warm the olive oil. Toss in the celery, carrots, and onion. Just a few minutes of simmering time should be enough to soften the veggies. After the minced garlic starts to release some aroma, add it to the pan and simmer for an additional minute.
2. Fill the slow cooker with all the ingredients.
3. Place the cooked veggies in the slow cooker.
4. Toss in the chopped tomatoes (with their juices), red kidney beans, cannellini beans, dried oregano, dried basil, dried thyme, rosemary, red pepper flakes (if used), salt, and black pepper. Additionally, you can add chicken or veggie broth. Combine all of the ingredients.

Prepare the Soup:

1. Once the vegetables are soft and the flavors have combined, simmer them covered for 6–8 hours on low or 3–4 hours on high.
2. Add Pasta: Stir in the tiny pasta about 30 minutes before the cooking time expires. Cover and cook the pasta until it's al dente.

Serve:

➢ After the soup is cooked and the pasta is soft, taste it, and, if necessary, adjust the seasoning.
➢ Garnish the heated Pasta e Fagioli with freshly cut parsley.
➢ Serve with grated Parmesan cheese for drizzling on top.

NOTE:

- ➤ Beans: Feel free to use a combination of cannellini and red kidney beans, but feel free to use whatever mix or kind you happen to have on hand.
- ➤ Toss in some elbow macaroni, ditalini, or small shells for the pasta in this soup. If you want your pasta al dente, prepare it separately according to the package guidelines.
- ➤ To your desire, add flavor and nutrients to your veggies. Alternatively, you might use bell peppers or chopped zucchini.
- ➤ You can modify the level of spiciness to your liking. The ideal amount of dried herbs and red pepper flakesto use is subjective and depends on personal taste.
- ➤ Assuring: upholdIf you seal any leftovers, you can keep them in the fridge for three days. Warm gently in a microwave or skillet over low heat until ready to serve.
- ➤ Fettuccine alfredo is such a great freezer dish. Wrap it in plastic and put it in the freezer for up to three months after it has cooled. Before cooking, let it defrost in the fridge for at least one night.

INGREDIENTS

- ❖ 4 bone-in, skin-on chicken thighs
- ❖ Salt and black pepper to taste
- ❖ 2 tablespoons all-purpose flour
- ❖ 2 tablespoons olive oil
- ❖ 1 onion, chopped
- ❖ 2 cloves garlic, minced
- ❖ 8 ounces mushrooms, sliced
- ❖ 1 can (14.5 oz) diced tomatoes, undrained
- ❖ 1/2 cup dry white wine
- ❖ 1/2 cup chicken broth
- ❖ 2 tablespoons tomato paste
- ❖ 1 teaspoon dried thyme
- ❖ 1 teaspoon dried parsley
- ❖ 1 bay leaf
- ❖ Chopped fresh parsley (for garnish)

INSTRUCTIONS

1. Season and flour the chicken: Sprinkle salt and black pepper on the thighs and lightly dust them with all-purpose flour.
2. To brown the chicken, place a skillet over medium-high heat with olive oil. The chicken thighs should be browned for three to four minutes on each side. When the chicken has browned, place it in the slow cooker.
3. Saute Aromatics: Add the minced garlic and diced onion to the same skillet. Simmer for three minutes or until tender.

Add the sliced mushrooms and simmer for five minutes or until they release their juices and begin to brown.

4. Add all ingredients to the slow cooker.
5. Add the chicken, sautéed onion, and mushroom combination to the slow cooker.
6. Add the chopped tomatoes (together with their liquids), dry white wine, chicken broth, tomato paste, dried parsley, dried thyme, and bay leaf to the slow cooker. Mix everything together.
7. Six to eight hours on low heat or three to four hours on high heat, covered, will cook the Chicken Chasseur. Thoroughly cooking and tenderizing the chicken is essential.

Serve:

- ➢ After cooking, remove the bay leaf.
- ➢ Garnish the hot Chicken Chasseur with finely chopped fresh parsley.

NOTE:

- ➢ Chicken: Bone-in, skin-on chicken thighs work best for this dish since they retain taste and moisture while cooking slowly. But you can also use chicken breasts.
- ➢ Mushrooms: This recipe works nicely with button or cremini mushrooms. Use the kind of mushrooms that you prefer.
- ➢ Wine: To enhance the sauce's flavor, use a dry white wine like Chardonnay or Sauvignon Blanc. If you would rather not use wine, you can use more chicken broth.

- The use of tomato paste thickens and enhances the flavor of the sauce. Feel free to omit it if you're short on it, but be prepared for a sauce that may lack flavor.
- Garnish: Fresh parsley adds a dash of color and freshness to the dish. The Chicken Chasseur can also be served over mashed potatoes, boiled rice, or crusty toast.

76. SLOW COOKER BEEF AND BEAN CHILI

INGREDIENTS

- ❖ 1 tablespoon olive oil
- ❖ 1 onion, chopped
- ❖ 2 cloves garlic, minced
- ❖ 1 pound ground beef (lean)
- ❖ 1 can (14.5 oz) diced tomatoes, undrained
- ❖ 1 can (15 oz) kidney beans, cleaned and drained
- ❖ 1 can (15 oz) black beans, cleaned and drained
- ❖ 1 can (6 oz) tomato paste
- ❖ 2 cups beef broth
- ❖ 1 tablespoon chili powder
- ❖ 1 teaspoon ground cumin
- ❖ 1 teaspoon paprika
- ❖ 1/2 teaspoon dried oregano
- ❖ 1/2 teaspoon ground coriander
- ❖ Salt and black pepper to taste
- ❖ Optional toppings: shredded cheese, sour cream, sliced green onions, chopped cilantro, diced avocado

INSTRUCTIONS

1. Saute Aromatics: Warm the olive oil in a skillet over medium heat. Add the minced garlic and diced onion. Cook for 3–4 minutes, or until tender.
2. Brown Ground Beef: Combine the ground beef, onions, and garlic in a skillet. Cook until the meat is browned and well done, breaking it up with a spoon as you go. Remove any extra fat.
3. Add all ingredients to the slow cooker.

4. Place the cooked mixture of meat into the slow cooker.
5. Add the diced tomatoes (together with their liquids), kidney beans, black beans, tomato paste, beef broth, ground cumin, paprika, dried oregano, ground coriander, salt, and black pepper to the slow cooker. Mix everything together.
6. Simmer the Chili: After the flavors have blended and the chili is thoroughly heated, cover and simmer on low for 6–8 hours or on high for 3–4 hours.

Serves:

- Taste the food after it's done cooking and make any necessary changes to the seasoning.
- You can top the hot Beef and Bean Chili with whatever you like, like sour cream, shredded cheese, chopped avocado, chopped cilantro, or sliced green onions.

NOTE:

➢ Ground Beef: To reduce unnecessary fat in this recipe, use lean ground beef. As a leaner substitute, you can alternatively use ground chicken or turkey.

➢ Beans: You can use any beans you choose or have on hand, but this recipe calls for a combination of kidney and black beans.

➢ Spices: Add or subtract chili powder and other spices as needed to suit your taste. For more heat, add more; for a softer flavor, minimize.

➢ Add your preferred toppings to your chili to make it uniquely yours. Popular options include diced avocado, chopped cilantro, sliced green onions, sour cream, and shredded cheese.

➤ Storage: Chili leftovers can be kept in the fridge for up to three days in an airtight container. Warm it up slowly in the microwave or on the stove before serving.

➤ Chili with beans and beef freezes well. Once it's completely cool, cut it up into pieces and put them in cases that can go in the freezer for up to three months. Thaw it in the fridge for at least one night before you prepare it.

INGREDIENTS

- ❖ 3-4 pound pork shoulder roast or pork loin roast
- ❖ Salt and black pepper to taste
- ❖ 2 tablespoons olive oil
- ❖ 1 onion, sliced
- ❖ 4 cloves garlic, minced
- ❖ 1 cup chicken broth or vegetable broth
- ❖ 1/2 cup of applesauce or cider
- ❖ 2 tablespoons soy sauce
- ❖ 2 tablespoons honey or maple syrup
- ❖ 1 tablespoon Dijon mustard
- ❖ 2 teaspoons dried thyme
- ❖ 2 teaspoons dried rosemary
- ❖ 2 teaspoons paprika
- ❖ 1 teaspoon garlic powder
- ❖ 1 teaspoon onion powder
- ❖ 1/2 teaspoon cayenne pepper (optional)

INSTRUCTIONS

1. Season the Pork Roast: Sprinkle a lot of salt and black pepper
2. on all sides of the pork roast.
3. Put olive oil in a big skillet and set it over medium-high heat. This will help the pork roast brown. For three to four minutes, or until browned, sear each side of the pork roast. Put the roast pig in the slow cooker
4. with the browned side facing down.

Prepare the sauce:

5. To make the sauce, put the chopped garlic, onion powder, garlic powder, chili pepper (if using), apple cider or juice, honey or maple syrup, Dijon mustard, dried thyme, and dried rosemary in a bowl.
6. Get the pork roast ready:
7. The sauce should be poured over the slow-cooked pork roast. Then, put the cut onions
8.   around the pork roast.
9. Simmer the pork with the lid on for 6–8 hours on low or 3–4 hours on high, or until it is soft and easy to cut with a fork.

To serve

- After the pork roast is done, put it on a cutting board and let it rest for a few minutes. Then you can slice or split it.
- Put onions and the pork roast's cooking juices on top of it, and serve it hot.

NOTE:

➢ Choose between a pork loin roast or a pork shoulder roast, which is also known as a pig butt, for this dish. Both cuts are great in a slow cooker; the meat gets soft and tasty after cooking for a long time.
➢ Searing: Searing the pork roast before putting it in the slow cooker makes it taste even better by caramelizing the outside of the meat.
➢ Sauce: The sauce gives the pork roast flavor and wetness as it cooks. Feel free to change the
➢ amount of sugar and spices to your liking.

- ➤ Carrots, potatoes, or bell peppers can be added to the slow cooker with the onions to make it taste and feel better.
- ➤ Storing: You can keep any extra pork roast and cooking liquids for up to three days in a container that won't let air in. Warm it up slowly in the microwave or on the stove before serving.
- ➤ Roast pork is a good food to freeze. Once it's completely cool, cut it up into pieces and put them in cases that can go in the freezer for up to three months. Thaw it in the fridge for at least one night before you prepare it.

INGREDIENTS

- ❖ 1 chicken legs that have been cut into bite-sized pieces and are boneless and skinless.
- ❖ 1 onion, finely chopped
- ❖ 4 cloves garlic, minced
- ❖ 1 tablespoon ginger, grated
- ❖ 1 can (14.5 oz) diced tomatoes, undrained
- ❖ 1/2 cup plain yogurt
- ❖ 1/4 cup butter, diced
- ❖ 1/4 cup heavy cream
- ❖ 2 tablespoons tomato paste
- ❖ 1 tablespoon garam masala
- ❖ 1 teaspoon ground cumin
- ❖ 1 teaspoon ground coriander
- ❖ 1 teaspoon ground turmeric
- ❖ 1/2 teaspoon paprika
- ❖ 1/4 teaspoon cayenne pepper (adjust to taste)
- ❖ Salt and black pepper to taste
- ❖ Fresh cilantro, chopped
- ❖ Cooked basmati rice or naan bread

1. To prepare the ingredients, cut the skinless, boneless chicken thighs into bite-sized pieces.
2. Finely chop the onion, mince the garlic, and grate the ginger.
3. Fill the slow cooker with all the ingredients.
4. In the slow cooker
5. , combine the chopped chicken thighs, finely chopped onion, minced garlic, grated ginger, diced tomatoes (with their juices), plain yogurt, diced butter, heavy cream, tomato paste, ground cumin, ground coriander, ground turmeric, paprika, cayenne pepper, salt, and black pepper. Combine all of the ingredients.
6. To make Butter Chicken,cook the chicken until it's tender and completely cooked. Then, cover it and simmer it on low for 7-8 hours or on high for 3-5 hours.
7. Before serving, taste the cooked Butter Chicken and adjust the seasoning if needed.
8. Add some freshly chopped cilantro, chopped finely, to the cooked Butter Chicken.
9. Serve with cooked basmati rice or warm naan bread.

NOTE:

➢ The ideal chicken thighs for this recipe are skinless and boneless because they keep their moisture and softness even after cooking at a slow temperature. Alternatively, you might use skinless, boneless chicken breasts.
➢ Tomatoes: Use fresh tomatoes when available, or, for convenience, use canned diced tomatoes.
➢ Spices: Garam masala is the main spice combination in this recipe, however you can adjust the quantity to your

preference. Reduce the amount of cayenne pepper for a gentler taste and increase it for additional heat.

➢ Creaminess: The combination of yogurt, butter, and heavy cream gives this butter chicken a rich, creamy texture. Use Greek yogurt and use less butter and heavy cream for a lighter version.

➢ Storage: You can keep any leftover butter chicken in the fridge for up to three days by placing it in an airtight container. Warm it up slowly in the microwave or on the stove before serving.

➢ How to Freeze Butter Chicken: It stays good in the freezer. First, let it cool completely. Then, split it up and put it in containers that can be frozen for up to three months. Before cooking it, let it thaw overnight in the fridge.

79. SLOW COOKER CABBAGE ROLL SOUP

INGREDIENTS

- ❖ 1 pound ground beef
- ❖ 1 onion, chopped
- ❖ 2 cloves garlic, minced
- ❖ 4 cups beef broth
- ❖ 1 can (14.5 oz) diced tomatoes, undrained
- ❖ 1 can (8 oz) tomato sauce
- ❖ 1/2 cup uncooked white rice
- ❖ 1 small head of cabbage, chopped
- ❖ 1 carrot, diced
- ❖ 1 celery stalk, diced
- ❖ 1 teaspoon dried oregano
- ❖ 1 teaspoon dried basil

- ❖ Salt and black pepper to taste
- ❖ Fresh parsley, chopped (for garnish)

INSTRUCTIONS

1. Break up the ground beef with a spoon as you brown it in a pan over medium-low heat. Get rid of fat.
2. Put everything in the slow cooker.
3. Ground beef in slow cooker.
4. Slow cooker ingredients should include diced carrot, celery, onion, garlic, tomato sauce, tomatoes (with liquids), cabbage, oregano, and basil. Combine ingredients.
5. Simmer soup: To tenderize rice and vegetables, cover and simmer for 7-8 hours on low or 3-5 hours on high.
6. Add salt and black pepper after cooking. After that, serve.
7. Once the cabbage roll soup is hot, add chopped parsley and mix it in.

NOTE:

- ➢ This soup can be made lighter with lean ground beef or turkey.
- ➢ Chop cabbage roughly into bite-sized pieces. For a finer texture, shred it instead of chopping.
- ➢ The soup cooks uncooked white rice with the other components. Cooked rice can be added at the end.
- ➢ Vegetables: Customize vegetables to taste. Diced potatoes or bell peppers can be added.
- ➢ Seasonings: Tailor to taste. Add dry herbs or spices for taste.

➤ Storage: Refrigerate leftover cabbage roll soup in an airtight container for three days. Reheat gently in the microwave or stovetop before serving.

➤ Cabbage roll soup freezes well. After cooling, portion and store in freezer-safe containers for up to 3 months. Thaw overnight in the fridge before heating.

INGREDIENTS

- ❖ 1 pound cremini mushrooms, sliced
- ❖ 1 onion, chopped
- ❖ 3 cloves garlic, minced
- ❖ 2 tablespoons olive oil
- ❖ 2 tablespoons all-purpose flour
- ❖ 2 cups vegetable broth or mushroom broth
- ❖ 1 tablespoon Worcestershire sauce
- ❖ 1 teaspoon Dijon mustard
- ❖ 1 teaspoon paprika
- ❖ 1/2 teaspoon dried thyme
- ❖ 1/2 teaspoon dried parsley
- ❖ Salt and black pepper to taste
- ❖ Half a cup of Greek yogurt or sour cream
- ❖ Cooked egg noodles or rice (for serving)
- ❖ Chopped fresh parsley (for garnish)

INSTRUCTIONS

1. Saute Onions and Mushrooms: Heat the olive oil in a skillet over medium-high heat. Add the chopped onion and sliced mushrooms. Simmer for five to seven minutes until the onions are tender and the mushrooms have turned golden brown. When aromatic, add the minced garlic and simmer for one more minute.
2. Dust the onions and mushrooms in the skillet with flour to make the sauce. Stir to coat evenly, then heat for one to two minutes.

3. Pour in the vegetable broth gradually, stirring constantly to avoid lumps. Stir in the Dijon mustard, paprika, dried thyme, parsley, Worcestershire sauce, salt, and black pepper. Mix everything together.
4. Switch to Slow Cooker:
5. Place the mixture of mushrooms into the slow cooker.
6. Cook: Cook, covered, for 4–5 hours on low or 2–3 hours on high, or until the sauce thickens and the flavors combine.
7. To finish and serve, add the Greek yogurt or sour cream and whisk until thoroughly mixed.
8. Warm up the Mushroom Stroganoff and serve it with rice or boiled egg noodles.
9. Add some freshly cut parsley on top before serving.

NOTE:

➢ Because of their deep flavor, cremini mushrooms yield the greatest results; however, you can also use white mushrooms or a combination of different varieties.
➢ Vegetable Broth: To add more flavor, use mushroom broth in place of vegetable broth.
➢ Sour Cream: To make this recipe lighter, you can substitute Greek yogurt for regular sour cream.
➢ Optional Additions: To increase taste and nutrition, you can add diced bell peppers, sliced carrots, or peas.
➢ Storage: Leftover mushroom stroganoff can be refrigerated for three days in an airtight container. Reheat gently in the microwave or stovetop before serving.
➢ Served frozen, stroganov with mushrooms is delicious. Cool fully, then separate and freeze in freezer-safe containers for 3 months. Thaw overnight in the fridge before heating.

INGREDIENTS

- ❖ 2 pounds of beef bones (such as marrow or knuckle bones)
- ❖ 1 onion, halved
- ❖ 3-inch piece of ginger, sliced and lightly smashed
- ❖ 4 cloves garlic, smashed
- ❖ 2 cinnamon sticks
- ❖ 4-star anise
- ❖ 4 cloves
- ❖ 1 cardamom pod
- ❖ 1 tablespoon coriander seeds
- ❖ 1 tablespoon fennel seeds
- ❖ 1 teaspoon black peppercorns
- ❖ 8 cups water
- ❖ 1 tablespoon fish sauce
- ❖ 1 tablespoon soy sauce
- ❖ 1 tablespoon sugar
- ❖ Salt, to taste
- ❖ 8 ounces rice noodles (pho noodles)
- ❖ 1 pound beef sirloin or flank steaka and thinly sliced
- ❖ Optional toppings: bean sprouts, thinly sliced onion, thinly sliced jalapeno peppers, fresh cilantro, Thai basil, lime wedges, hoisin sauce, sriracha sauce

INSTRUCTIONS

1. Start the broth with beef bones in the slow cooker. Add water, coriander, fennel, cloves, onion halves, ginger slices, cinnamon sticks, star anise, cloves, cardamom pod, and black peppercorns.
2. Prepare Broth:
3. When the soup is rich and flavorful, cover and boil for 8–10 hours on low or 4–6 hours on high.
4. Strain soup: After the soup simmers, remove the meat bones and aromatics from the slow cooker. Remove particulates from broth with cheesecloth or a fine mesh filter. Get rid of solids.
5. Return strained broth to slow cooker and season. Add sugar, soy, and fish sauce. Salt to taste.
6. Noodles and Beef: Cook rice noodles according to the package guidelines until al dente. Run cold water after emptying.
7. Thinly slice flank steak or beef sirloin.

To present:

- Distribute the cooked rice noodles among serving dishes. Add some raw beef slices on top.
- As you ladle the hot broth over the noodles and steak, make sure the meat is completely covered. The heated broth will cook the beef slices.
- Serve the heated Beef Pho with optional toppings like lime wedges, fresh cilantro, Thai basil, thinly sliced onion, thinly sliced jalapeño peppers, bean sprouts, and hoisin and sriracha sauce.

NOTE:

- ➢ Beef Bones: The savory broth for Beef Pho is typically made with marrow or knuckle bones. Most grocery stores and butcher shops carry them.
- ➢ Aromatics: The addition of spices, onion, ginger, and garlic deepens the broth's flavor. The quantity of spices can be changed to suit your personal preferences.
- ➢ Noodles: Rice noodles, sometimes referred to as pho noodles, are the staple of beef pho. Before serving, cook them individually as directed on the package.
- ➢ Beef: Thinly sliced raw beef is added to the heated broth just before serving. The beef slices in the boiling broth will be cooked to the proper doneness.
- ➢ Spice up your Beef Pho with bean sprouts, onion, jalapeño peppers, lime wedges, cilantro, Thai basil, and hoisin and sriracha sauce.
- ➢ Storage: You may keep any leftover noodles and broth separate in the fridge for up to three days. Before serving, reheat the broth and prepare fresh noodles as needed.
- ➢ Frozen beef pho soup is good. Divide it and store it in freezer-safe containers for up to three months after cooling. Let it thaw overnight in the fridge before heating.

82. COOKER PORK POSOLE

INGREDIENTS

- ❖ 2 pounds pork shoulder, trimmed of excess fat and cut into chunks
- ❖ Salt and black pepper to taste
- ❖ 1 tablespoon olive oil
- ❖ 1 onion, chopped
- ❖ 4 cloves garlic, minced
- ❖ 2 teaspoons ground cumin
- ❖ 1 teaspoon dried oregano
- ❖ 1 teaspoon smoked paprika
- ❖ 1/2 teaspoon ground coriander
- ❖ 1/2 teaspoon chili powder
- ❖ 2 cans (15 oz each) of hominy, drained and rinsed
- ❖ 1 can (14.5 oz) diced tomatoes, undrained
- ❖ 4 cups chicken broth
- ❖ Juice of 2 limes
- ❖ Salt and black pepper to taste
- ❖ Optional toppings: sliced radishes, chopped cilantro, sliced avocado, lime wedges, shredded cabbage, diced onion, hot sauce

INSTRUCTIONS

1. Brown the pork shoulder chunks with salt and pepper.The olive oil should be warmed in a skillet over medium-high heat just before serving. If you need to cook the meat in batches, that's okay. Move the beef from the skillet to the slow cooker after browning it in a medium-sized skillet.
2. Sautée Aromatiques: Simmer the chopped onion in the same skillet for 5 minutes to soften. Stir in chili powder, ground coriander, smoked paprika, dried oregano, minced garlic, and cumin. Simmer until fragrant, another minute.
3. Put everything in the slow cooker.
4. After browning the pork, add the sautéed onion and spices to the slow cooker.
5. Drain and rinse hominy and add to slow cooker with diced tomatoes and chicken broth. Combine everything.
6. Once the pig is soft and the flavors have combined, cover and cook the posole for 6–8 hours on low or 3–4 hours on high.
7. After cooking, taste the lime juice and add salt and black pepper to serve.

Top hot pork posole with diced onion, shredded cabbage, lime wedges, chopped cilantro, sliced radishes, and spicy sauce.

NOTE:

- ➤ Pork Shoulder: Slow cooking brings out pork shoulder's natural tenderness and flavor. If preferred, you can also use pork loin or butt.
- ➤ Hominy: Hominy gives the posole a distinct flavor and texture. Check the Latin foods area of your grocery store for canned hominy.
- ➤ Spices: You can vary the quantity of spices to suit your tastes. If you want a softer taste, you can leave out the chili powder or add more for more excellent heat.
- ➤ To personalize your pork posole, you can add a choice of toppings, such as diced onion, shredded cabbage, lime wedges, chopped cilantro, sliced avocado, and sliced radishes.
- ➤ Storage: Any leftover pork posole can be stored in an airtight container in the refrigerator forp any leftover po Before serving, gently reheat in the microwave or on the stove.
- ➤ Pork posole freezes well. Divide it and store it in freezer-safe containers for up to three months after cooling. Let it thaw overnight in the fridge before heating.

INGREDIENTS

- ❖ 1 tablespoon olive oil
- ❖ 1 onion, chopped
- ❖ 2 carrots, diced
- ❖ 2 celery stalks, diced
- ❖ 3 cloves garlic, minced
- ❖ 1 pound Italian sausage, casings removed
- ❖ One cup of washed and drained dried brown lentils
- ❖ 1 can (14.5 oz) diced tomatoes, undrained
- ❖ 4 cups chicken broth or vegetable broth
- ❖ 1 teaspoon dried thyme
- ❖ 1 teaspoon dried oregano
- ❖ 1 bay leaf
- ❖ Salt and black pepper to taste
- ❖ Fresh parsley, chopped (for garnish)

INSTRUCTIONS

1. **To sauté aromatics**, heat olive oil in a skillet on medium. Add chopped carrots, celery, and onion. Simmer 5 minutes until soft. When aromatic, add minced garlic and cook another minute. After cooking, add veggies to slow cooker.
2. **Br**eak Italian sausage with a spoon in the skillet to brown. Cook and brown well. Add cooked sausage to the slow cooker with fat removed.
3. Put everything in slow cooker.
4. Drain and rinse brown lentils. Put chopped tomatoes, juices, dried oregano, thyme, and bay leaf in the slow cooker. Mix everything.

5. Boil stew on low for 6-8 hours or high for 3-4 hours

when lentils are soft and flavors mingle.

Add fresh parsley to hot sausage-lentil stew.

NOTE:

- ➢ Use mild or hot Italian sausage to taste. Use turkey or chicken sausage to lighten.
- ➢ Brown lentils add heartiness and shape to the stew. Wash and drain before putting in the slow cooker.
- ➢ Vegetables: Customize the stew's vegetables. You can add diced potatoes, spinach, or bell peppers for flavor and nutrients.
- ➢ Broth: Build the stew with vegetable or chicken broth. Use low-sodium broth to balance the stew's saltiness.
- ➢ Herbs: Dried thyme, oregano, and bay leaf flavor the stew. Adjust the herb quantity to your liking.
- ➢ Storage: Refrigerate leftover sausage and lentil stew for three days in an airtight container. Reheat gently in microwave or stove before serving.
- ➢ Lentil-sausage stew freezes well. Divide it and store it in freezer-safe containers for up to three months after cooling. Let it thaw overnight in the fridge before heating.

84. SLOW COOKER CHICKEN MARBELLA

INGREDIENTS:

- ❖ 4-6 bone-in, skin-on chicken thighs
- ❖ 4-6 bone-in, skin-on chicken drumsticks
- ❖ Salt and pepper to taste
- ❖ 1/2 cup pitted prunes
- ❖ 1/4 cup pitted green olives
- ❖ 1/4 cup capers, drained
- ❖ 4 cloves garlic, minced
- ❖ 2 tablespoons dried oregano
- ❖ 1/4 cup red wine vinegar
- ❖ 1/4 cup olive oil
- ❖ 1/2 cup brown sugar
- ❖ 1 cup chicken broth
- ❖ Finely cut 1/4 cup fresh parsley for garnish.
- ❖ Cooked couscous or rice (for serving)

INSTRUCTIONS:

1. Chicken Seasoning: Rub chicken thighs and drumsticks with salt and pepper to taste.
2. Prepare the slow cooker: Place chicken chunks in slow cooker.
3. In a separate bowl, mix prunes, capers, green olives, minced garlic, dried oregano, red wine vinegar, olive oil, brown sugar, and chicken broth.
4. Pour Marinade on Chicken: To coat the slow cooker chicken pieces evenly, pour the marinade mixture.
5. Cover and simmer chicken on low for 6–8 hours or high for 3–4 hours until tender and done.

6. Sprinkle finely chopped parsley over cooked Chicken Marbella. Serve with couscous or rice.

NOTE:

- ➢ Chicken: Use skin-on and bone-in drumsticks and thighs for this recipe. If preferable, use chicken breasts; cook longer because they cook faster.
- ➢ Chicken Marbella's unique flavor comes from acidic olives and sweet prunes. You can adjust olive and prune amounts to taste.
- ➢ Chicken releases marinade flavor as it cooks. Apply marinade evenly to chicken pieces for best results.
- ➢ Cooking Liquid: poultry broth makes a wonderful sauce and keeps poultry moist. After cooking the chicken, take it from the slow cooker and reduce the sauce on the stovetop until desired.
- ➢ Parsley garnishes the dish with color and freshness. Add extra capers and olives if desired.
- ➢ Serve Chicken Marbella over rice or couscous to soak up the sauce.
- ➢ Leftover chicken Marbella can be refrigerated for three days in an airtight container. Reheat gently in the microwave or stove before serving.

INGREDIENT:

- ❖ 1 pound Great Northern or Cannellini dried white beans, soaking overnight and drained
- ❖ 4 duck legs confit (or substitute with duck breasts)
- ❖ 4 pork sausages (such as Toulouse sausage or other flavorful sausage), sliced
- ❖ 1 onion, chopped
- ❖ 4 cloves garlic, minced
- ❖ 2 carrots, diced
- ❖ 2 celery stalks, diced
- ❖ 4 cups chicken broth or vegetable broth
- ❖ 1 can (14.5 oz) diced tomatoes, undrained
- ❖ 1 bay leaf
- ❖ 2 fresh or 1 teaspoon dried thyme sprigs
- ❖ Salt and black pepper to taste
- ❖ 1 cup breadcrumbs
- ❖ Chopped fresh parsley (for garnish)

INSTRUCTIONS:

1. Prepare Ingredients: Soak dry white beans overnight. Drain and rinse beans before using. Take duck legs confit out of the fat and dry with paper towels.
2. Layer Ingredients in Slow Cooker: Layer soaked and drained white beans, duck legs confit, sliced pork sausages, chopped onion, minced garlic, diced carrots, and diced celery.
3. Pour in liquid and seasonings. Pour chicken or veggie broth over slow cooker items. Add chopped tomatoes,

juices, bay leaf, and fresh or dried thyme sprigs; season with salt and black pepper to taste.

4. Cook: Cover and simmer on low for 6-8 hours or high for 3-4 hours to tenderize beans and blend flavors.
5. Breadcrumbs: Toast breadcrumbs in a separate skillet over medium heat until golden brown and crispy.
6. Finish and Serve: Remove the slow cooker bay leaf and thyme sprigs after cooking. Add salt and black pepper to taste. Serve cassoulet hot with chopped fresh parsley and toasted breadcrumbs.

NOTES:

➢ Soak dry white beans overnight to soften and shorten cooking time. Use canned white beans but alter the cooking time if you're short on time.
➢ Meat: Duck confit, pig sausages, and pork shoulder are common in cassoulet. Change the meat to your liking.
➢ Onion, garlic, carrots, and celery flavor and aromatize Cassoulet. Add chopped tomatoes or diced bell peppers for flavor.
➢ Toasted breadcrumbs give Cassoulet a crispy top. Fresh breadcrumbs or omission are also options.
➢ Garnish: Chopped fresh parsley brightens the dish. Additional thyme leaves can be garnished.
➢ Leftover Cassoulet can be refrigerated for 3 days in an airtight container. Reheat gently on the burner or microwave before serving.

86. SLOW COOKER TERIYAKI CHICKEN

INGREDIENT:

- ❖ 1.5 lbs boneless and skinless chicken thighs (or breast) cut into bite-sized pieces
- ❖ 1/2 cup low-sodium soy sauce
- ❖ 1/4 cup honey
- ❖ 2 tablespoons rice vinegar
- ❖ 2 cloves garlic, minced
- ❖ 1 teaspoon grated fresh ginger
- ❖ 1 tablespoon cornstarch
- ❖ 1 tablespoon water
- ❖ Optional garnish: sliced green onions, sesame seeds, chopped cilantro

INSTRUCTIONS:

1. Mix low-sodium soy sauce, honey, rice vinegar, garlic, and ginger in a bowl. Mix.
2. Chicken should be coated before slow cooking. Apply homemade teriyaki sauce to chicken.
3. Prepare food: After the chicken is tender, cover and cook on low for 4–5 hours or high for 2–3 hours.
4. Optional Sauce Thickness: Mix cornstarch and water in a small bowl. Mix the slurry with the chicken and sauce in the slow cooker. Simmer sauce on high for 15–20 minutes to thicken.
1. Hot Teriyaki Chicken can be topped with cilantro, sesame seeds, or green onions. Add hot noodles or rice.

NOTE:

- ➤ This meal works well with boneless, skinless chicken thighs. The flavor and juicy texture will linger after extended cooking. Chicken breastworks too.
- ➤ Use low-sodium soy sauce to cut salt.
- ➤ Sweeten honey to taste.
- ➤ A cornstarch slurry thickens the sauce at the end. Thin the sauce to skip this step.
- ➤ Chopped cilantro, sesame seeds, and green onions provide crunch and flavor. Add whatever you want.
- ➤ Stay safe:Sealable Refrigerate Teriyaki Chicken for three days. Prior to consumption, reheat it in a microwave or oven.
- ➤ Great Teriyaki Chicken Freezes. Keep cooled servings in freezer-safe containers for three months. Thaw overnight in the fridge before cooking.

INGREDIENTS:

- ❖ 2 pounds beef chuck roast, thinly sliced
- ❖ 1/2 cup low-sodium soy sauce
- ❖ 1/4 cup brown sugar
- ❖ 4 cloves garlic, minced
- ❖ 1 tablespoon sesame oil
- ❖ 1 tablespoon grated fresh ginger
- ❖ 2 tablespoons rice vinegar
- ❖ 1 tablespoon sriracha sauce (adjust to taste)
- ❖ To make the garnish, you'll need 2 chopped green onions.
- ❖ 1/3 cup cornstarch
- ❖ 1 tablespoon water
- ❖ Optional garnish: sesame seeds, sliced green onions, chopped cilantro

INSTRUCTIONS:

1. Mix all sauce ingredients in a bowl. Stir in rice vinegar, chopped green onions, garlic, sesame oil, fresh ginger, and sriracha. Finish with minced garlic.
2. Before slow cooking, slice and sauce beef chuck roast. Pour your own sauce over the
3. meat, covering it well.
4. Make meals: To tenderize and cook beef, simmer on low 6-8 hours or high 3-4 hours.
5. Set aside cornstarch-water slurry. This optional step thickens sauce. Combine slurry, sauce, and slow-cooked beef. Simmer covered for 15–20 minutes to thicken sauce.

6. Chopped cilantro and green onions replace sesame seeds on hot Korean beef. Good with heated noodles or rice.

NOTE:

- ➢ Long cooking tenderizes and flavors chuck roast, so this recipe is ideal. Use flank or sirloin steaks as desired.
- ➢ Use low-sodium soy sauce to minimize saltiness.
- ➢ Add additional brown sugar for a sweeter recipe.
- ➢ Use as much Sriracha as your spicy tolerance allows. Use gochujang, a Korean chili paste, to boost flavor.
- ➢ For flavor and crunch, add chopped cilantro, green onions, and sesame seeds. Top it with your favorite toppings to customize.
- ➢ You can refrigerate leftover Korean beef for three days in an airtight container. Reheat it slightly in the oven or microwave before serving.
- ➢ I like Korean frozen beef. Divide the cooled mixture into servings and store in freezer-safe containers for three months. Thaw overnight in the fridge before cooking.

88. SLOW COOKER POZOLE ROJO

INGREDIENTS:

- ❖ 2 pounds pork shoulder, cut into chunks
- ❖ 1 onion, chopped
- ❖ 4 cloves garlic, minced
- ❖ 2 dried ancho chilies, stems, and seeds removed
- ❖ 2 dried guajillo chilies, stems, and seeds removed
- ❖ 1 can (28 oz) hominy, drained and rinsed
- ❖ 6 cups chicken broth
- ❖ 1 teaspoon dried oregano
- ❖ 1 teaspoon ground cumin
- ❖ Salt and pepper to taste
- ❖ Optional toppings: shredded cabbage, sliced radishes, chopped cilantro, diced onion, lime wedges, oregano, avocado slices, tortilla chips

INSTRUCTIONS:

1. In a bowl, combine the dried guajillo and ancho chilies. Set aside. To make them soft, boil some water and cover them; soak for 20 to 30 minutes. Remove the chiles from the liquid after they have softened, and discard the soaking water.
2. Process or blend the Soaked and Drained Chilies, Minced Garlic, Onion, and Chicken Stock. Once soft, blend until smooth; add broth as needed.
3. Go ahead and put everything in the slow cooker. Load the slow cooker with the pork shoulder cubes. Spread the chile mixture over the pork. Stir in the hominy that has been washed and drained, along with any remaining chicken

stock, ground cumin, dried oregano, salt, and pepper. Blend all of the ingredients.

4. Prepare food: After the pork is soft, cover and simmer on low for 8–10 hours or high for 4–6 hours.
5. Double-fork-shred meat in the slow cooker.

Serve:

- Present the Pozole Rojo hot, accompanied by tortilla chips, avocado slices, chopped cilantro, diced onion, lime wedges, shredded cabbage, and sliced radishes.

NOTES:

➢ Pork Shoulder: Slow cooking makes pork shoulder soft and delicious, making it perfect for Pozole Rojo. If preferred, you can also use pork loin or butt.

➢ Chilies: Adding ancho and guajillo chilies enhances the pozole Rojo's rich red color and flavor. If you want your pozole hotter, add more chiles, like arbol or pasilla.

➢ Hominy: Hominy gives the pozole body and texture. Check the Latin foods area of your grocery store for canned hominy.

➢ To personalize your Pozole Rojo, add shredded cabbage, sliced radishes, chopped cilantro, diced onion, lime wedges, dry oregano, avocado slices, and tortilla chips.

➢ Storage: Any leftover pozole rojo can be kept in an airtight container in the refrigerator for up to three days. Warm it up a little in the oven or microwave before serving.

➢ Freezing Pozole Rojo is a breeze. Split it into servings and put each one in a freezer-safe container; after it has cooled completely, you can keep them for up to three months. Put it in the fridge to thaw overnight before you cook it.

89. SLOW COOKER GREEK LEMON CHICKEN SOUP (AVGOLEMONO)

INGREDIENTS:

- ❖ 4 cups chicken broth
- ❖ 1 pound boneless, skinless chicken breasts
- ❖ 1/2 cup uncooked long-grain white rice
- ❖ 3 eggs
- ❖ Juice of 2-3 lemons (about 1/2 cup)
- ❖ Salt and pepper to taste
- ❖ Fresh dill or parsley, chopped (for garnish)
- ❖ Lemon slices (for garnish)

INSTRUCTIONS:

1. Pour in half of the chicken broth before adding the rest of the ingredients to the slow cooker. Mix the deboned and skinned chicken breasts with the raw rice. Season to taste with salt and pepper.
2. Get the slow cooker started by adding half of the chicken stock. Next, combine all of the remaining components. Mix the deboned and skinned chicken breasts with the raw rice.
3. Adjust salt and pepper to taste.
4. Cover and boil on medium for 6-8 hours (or 3-4 on high) until chicken and rice are almost done.
5. After slow cooking, shred chicken breasts using two forks. Put shredded chicken back in slow cooker.
6. Avgolemono sauce prep. Eggs and lemon juice in basin.
7. To temper the eggs, carefully pour in approximately a cup of the hot broth while whisking frequently to prevent

curdling. Whisk in the lemon mixture before putting to the slow cooker.

8. When you return the tempered egg and lemon combination to the slow cooker, add the avgolemono sauce to the broth. Incorporate the saucewhile whisking continually.

9. If you feel like it's missing anything, season with more salt and pepper.

10. Each guest should have a bowl of the Greek Lemon Chicken Soup. Serve topped with thinly sliced lemons and freshly chopped dill or parsley.

NOTES:

> The chicken broth for this dish can be made from scratch or bought from the shop. To avoid an overly salty soup, use low-sodium chicken stock if you must buy it at the store.

> If possible, use skinless, boneless breasts instead of thighs when cooking the chicken.

> Although tiny pastas like orzo work just as well i

> n Avgolemono soup, long-grain white rice is the traditional ingredient.

> The avgolemono sauce is a thickening and flavor-enhancing mixture of eggs and lemon juice.

> To finish off the soup, garnish it with lemon slices and some fresh dill or parsley for a zesty flavor. A pinch of black pepper can also be used for flavor.

> If you store any leftover Greek Lemon Chicken Soup in an airtight container, you can enjoy it for three days in the fridge. Warm it up a little in the oven or microwave before serving.

90. SLOW COOKER CHICKEN AND WHITE BEAN CHILI

INGREDIENTS:

- ❖ 1 pound boneless, skinless chicken breasts
- ❖ Two 15-ounce washed and drained white beans (navy or cannellini beans)
- ❖ 1 onion, chopped
- ❖ 2 cloves garlic, minced
- ❖ 1 can (4 oz) diced green chilies
- ❖ 1 teaspoon ground cumin
- ❖ 1 teaspoon dried oregano
- ❖ 1/2 teaspoon ground coriander
- ❖ 1/2 teaspoon paprika
- ❖ 1/4 teaspoon cayenne pepper (optional for heat)
- ❖ 4 cups chicken broth
- ❖ 1 cup frozen corn kernels
- ❖ Salt and black pepper to taste
- ❖ Optional toppings: chopped fresh cilantro, sliced green onions, shredded cheese, sour cream, avocado slices, lime wedges, tortilla chips

1. After deboning the chicken breasts, put them in a slow cooker. All of the parts must be mixed together. The following ingredients should be mixed in a bowl: garlic, green chilies, onion, cumin, coriander, dried oregano, paprika, and maybe cayenne pepper. Combine by stirring. After removing excess water, give the white beansa good rinsing.

2. Pour the chicken stock over the chicken once you've put it in the slow cooker.

3. Cook the chicken for three to four hours, or until it reaches tenderness, after boiling. Reduce heat to a simmer.

4. Once taken out of the slow cooker, shred the cooked chicken breasts using two forks. Next, put the shredded chicken back into the slow cooker.

5. Just throw some frozen corn kernels into a slow cooker, and you're good to go. Mix everything together.

6. Add salt and black pepper, then taste.

Serve:

- Top the hot Chicken and White Bean Chili with avocado slices, lime wedges, shredded cheese, sour cream, and finely chopped fresh cilantro. Provide tortilla chips with the chili so they can be crumbled or dipped.

NOTE:

- Chicken:
- Instead of using skinless, boneless chicken breasts, you have the option to utilize chicken thighs. Make sure to remove the bones before shredding bone-in chicken.
- White Beans: You may use any white beans you have on hand for this chili, but cannellini or navy beans are great.
- Spices: You can vary the quantity of spices to suit your tastes. If you want a milder chili, leave off the cayenne pepper or add more for more excellent heat.
- Corn: The chili benefits from the sweetness and texture of frozen corn. However, you can also use fresh or canned corn kernels.
- You can add special touches to your Chicken and White Bean Chili, such as shredded cheese, sour cream, avocado slices, lime wedges, chopped fresh cilantro, and sliced green onions.
- Storage: Chili leftovers can be kept in the fridge for up to three days in an airtight container. Warm it up little in the oven or microwave before serving.

91. SLOW COOKER QUINOA AND BLACK BEAN STEW

INGREDIENTS:

- ❖ 1 cup quinoa, rinsed
- ❖ After draining and rinsing, use two 15-ounce cans of black beans.
- ❖ 1 chopped onion
- ❖ 2 cloves garlic, minced
- ❖ 2 carrots, diced
- ❖ 2 celery stalks, diced
- ❖ 1 bell pepper, diced (any color)
- ❖ 1 can (14.5 oz) diced tomatoes, undrained
- ❖ 4 cups vegetable broth or chicken broth
- ❖ 1 teaspoon ground cumin
- ❖ 1 teaspoon chili powder
- ❖ 1/2 teaspoon paprika
- ❖ Salt and black pepper to taste
- ❖ Optional toppings: chopped fresh cilantro, diced avocado, sour cream, shredded cheese, lime wedges

INSTRUCTIONS:

1. In a slow cooker, mix together the following ingredients: quinoa that has been rinsed, black beans, diced tomatoes (with their fluids), diced bell pepper, chopped celery, diced carrots, diced celery, diced onion, minced garlic, and ground cumin. Toss in some ground chili powder, paprika, cumin, salt, and black pepper.
2. After the vegetables and quinoa are tender, cover and cook for 6-8 hours on low or 3-4 hours on high.

3. Seasonality: Add more salt and black pepper according to your taste.

Serve:

- Bowls should be filled with the
- quinoa and black bean stew. For garnish, you can add shredded cheese, sliced avocado, chopped fresh cilantro, sour cream, and lime juice, if you like.

NOTE:

➢ Before placing the quinoa in the slow cooker, give it a good rinse to get rid of any bitter texture.

➢ You can also use cooke

➢ d dried black beans instead of canned beans if you like. First, wash and drain them, and then put them in the slow cooker.

➢ To make the stew your own, feel free to change up the vegetables. For added taste and nutrition, try adding diced potatoes, corn kernels, or zucchini.

➢ Broth: If you're not vegetarian, you can use chicken broth; if you are, you can use vegetable broth.

➢ Seasonings: Adjust the amount of seasonings according to your preference. Swap out or increase the amount of chili powder for a hotter stew.

➢ To make your Quinoa and Black Bean Stew extra special, you may garnish it with sliced avocado, sour cream, shredded cheese, wedges of lime, and chopped fresh cilantro.

➢ Preserving: If you make extra stew, cover it tightly and keep it in the fridge for three days. Warm it up a little in the oven or microwave before serving.

INGREDIENTS:

- ❖ Chop one pound of skinless, boneless chicken thighs into bite-sized pieces. Substitute tofu or vegetables for the chicken if you're a vegetarian.
- ❖ One 13.5-ounce can of fresh coconut milk
- ❖ Use two or three teaspoons of Thai red curry paste
- ❖ , depending on your preference.
- ❖ Two bell peppers, roughly diced
- ❖ , and one thinly sliced onion
- ❖ Delicately cut mushrooms in a spoonfull
- ❖ One cup of diced
- ❖ potatoes and one cup of chopped carrots
- ❖ Substitute two tablespoons of soy sauce for the fish sauce to make it vegetarian.
- ❖ After tasting, add two teaspoons of brown sugar.
- ❖ 2 kaffir lime leaves (optional)
- ❖ 1 tablespoon grated fresh ginger
- ❖ 2 cloves garlic, minced
- ❖ Juice of 1 lime
- ❖ Salt and pepper to taste
- ❖ Fresh cilantro leaves, chopped (for garnish)
- ❖ Cooked rice or noodles for serving

INSTRUCTIONS:

1. Slow cooker items should include grated fresh ginger, minced garlic, lime juice, fish sauce (or soy sauce), brown sugar, sliced onion, bell peppers, mushrooms, carrots, potatoes, and coconut milk. Mix everything.

2. Add Chicken: Cover bite-sized chicken thighs with curry in the slow cooker.
3. After the chicken and vegetables are soft, cover and simmer on low for 6–8 hours or high for 3–4 hours.
4. Add lime juice, brown sugar, salt, and pepper to taste in the curry.

Serve

- Thai Red Curry hot with finely chopped fresh cilantro. With rice or noodles.

NOTES:

- ➤ Chicken: Boneless, skinless thighs are ideal, but bone-in chunks or breast work too. You can make it vegetarian with tofu or veggies.
- ➤ Fatty coconut milk produces a delicious meal. A milder curry with half the coconut milk may need more cream.
- ➤ Thai red curry paste: Consider your hot meal tolerance when measuring paste. Start with two tablespoons and add more for hotter curry.
- ➤ Customize the curry's vegetables. Add spinach, snap peas, baby corn, or bamboo shoots.
- ➤ Fish Sauce: Deepen vegetarian curry flavor with soy sauce instead of fish sauce.
- ➤ Coriander leaves add freshness. Top with chopped peanuts or red chili peppers for flavor and texture.

➢ Storage: KeepRefrigerate Thai red curry leftovers for three days in an airtight container. Reheat gently in microwave or stove before serving.

93. SLOW COOKER CAJUN CHICKEN PASTA

INGREDIENTS:

- ❖ A pound of bite-sized, boneless, skinless chicken breasts
- ❖ 1 onion, diced
- ❖ 1 bell pepper, diced
- ❖ 2 cloves garlic, minced
- ❖ 1 can (14.5 oz) diced tomatoes, undrained
- ❖ 1 cup chicken broth
- ❖ 1 cup heavy cream
- ❖ 2 teaspoons Cajun seasoning
- ❖ 1 teaspoon paprika
- ❖ 1/2 teaspoon dried thyme
- ❖ 1/2 teaspoon dried oregano
- ❖ Salt and pepper to taste
- ❖ 8 oz penne pasta (or your preferred pasta shape)
- ❖ 1/2 cup grated Parmesan cheese
- ❖ Chopped fresh parsley for garnish

INSTRUCTIONS:

1. In a slow cooker, combine chicken stock, heavy cream, diced tomatoes (with juices), diced onion, diced bell pepper, minced garlic, dried thyme, dried oregano, paprika, Cajun spice, salt, and pepper. Give everything a good stir.
2. Simmer the chicken covered for 6–8 hours on low or 3–4 hours on high after it is tender.
3. Pasta Fits Here: Stir in raw penne 30 minutes before serving. Cover and cook pasta al dente.

4. Finally, stir cooked pasta with grated Parmesan cheese to melt and thicken.
5. Sprinkle chopped parsley over heated Cajun Chicken Pasta

NOTE:

- ➢ Chicken: Skinless, boneless chicken breasts are ideal for this recipe. But you could also use the thighs of chicken. For a spicier version, use sausage that has been spiced with Cajun spices or add extra Cajun spice.
- ➢ Vegetables: The spaghetti's flavor and texture come from chopped onions and bell peppers. Other vegetables, such as sliced mushrooms or diced tomatoes, can be added.
- ➢ Cajun seasoning: You can make your own at home by combining paprika, cayenne pepper, onion powder, garlic powder, and other spices, or you can buy it from the market.
- ➢ Pasta: Any pasta will work for this Cajun Chicken Pasta recipe, though penne is the typical option. As instructed on the packaging, adjust the cooking time.
- ➢ Cream: Rich, creamy sauces are enhanced by heavy cream. For a lighter version, you may use whole milk or half-and-half, but the sauce might need to have more flavor.
- ➢ Garnish: A dash of fresh parsley gives the food some color and vibrancy. As a garnish, feel free to top with extra grated Parmesan cheese.
- ➢ Storage: You may keep any leftover Cajun Chicken Pasta for up to three days in the refrigerator in an airtight container. Reheat gently in the microwave or stovetop before serving.

94. SLOW COOKER FISH STEW

INGREDIENTS:

- ❖ 1 pound white fish fillets , cut into chunks
- ❖ 1 onion, diced
- ❖ 2 cloves garlic, minced
- ❖ 2 carrots, diced
- ❖ 2 celery stalks, diced
- ❖ 1 bell pepper, diced
- ❖ 1 can (14.5 oz) diced tomatoes, undrained
- ❖ 3 cups fish or seafood broth (or vegetable broth)
- ❖ 1/2 cup dry white wine (optional)
- ❖ 1 teaspoon dried thyme
- ❖ 1 teaspoon dried oregano
- ❖ 1 bay leaf
- ❖ Salt and pepper to taste
- ❖ 1/4 cup all-purpose flour
- ❖ 1/4 cup water
- ❖ Chopped fresh parsley for garnish
- ❖ Crusty bread or rice for serving

INSTRUCTIONS:

1. Add all ingredients to the slow cooker. Diced onion, minced garlic, chopped celery, chopped carrots, chopped bell pepper, chopped tomatoes (with their juices), fish or seafood broth, dry white wine (if needed), dried thyme, dried oregano, bay leaf, salt, and pepper should all be combined in the slow cooker. Mix everything.
2. Simmer: Cover and simmer on low for 6–8 hours or on high for 3–4 hours until the vegetables are soft.

3. Condense Stew: To form a slurry, combine the all-purpose flour and water in a small basin and whisk until smooth. Stir the slurry in the slow cooker until thoroughly mixed. Simmer the stew for a half hour on high or until it has somewhat thickened.
4. Fish Addition: Add the white fish fillet chunks to the slow cooker and stir them gently so they are incorporated into the stew. Fry the fish on low for a further 15 to 20 minutes, covered, or until it is cooked through and readily flakes with a fork.

Serve:

- Top the hot fish stew with freshly chopped parsley. For a full dinner, serve over rice or with crusty bread.

NOTES:

> Fish: Haddocks, halibut, cod, or tilapia are just a few examples of white fish fillets that you can utilize. To make sure the fish cooks evenly in the stew, chop it into chunks.
> vegetables: Chopped bell pepper, celery, carrots, onions, and garlic provide the stew's taste and texture. Other veggies can be included, such as spinach, potatoes, or zucchini.
> Broth: To bring out the taste of the seafood, use fish or seafood broth as the stew's foundation. If not available, you can use chicken or vegetarian broth instead.
> Wine: Dry white wine gives the stew more flavor depth, but you can leave it out if you'd like.
> Thickening: The stew is thickened by the mixture of water and all-purpose flour. Cornstarch can be used in place of flour for a gluten-free alternative.

➢ Garnish: Finely chopped fresh parsley gives the dish a vibrant look. Add more freshly cracked black pepper or a squeeze of lemon juice as a garnish if preferred.
➢ Storage: Any leftover fish stew can be stored in an airtight container forp any leftover fi. Before serving, slowly reheat over the stove.

INGREDIENTS:

- ❖ 1-pound boneless, skinless chicken breasts sliced into bite-sized pieces
- ❖ 1 onion, thinly sliced
- ❖ 2 bell peppers, thinly sliced (any color)
- ❖ 1 cup chicken broth
- ❖ 1/2 cup creamy peanut butter
- ❖ 1/4 cup soy sauce
- ❖ 2 tablespoons honey
- ❖ 2 tablespoons rice vinegar
- ❖ 2 cloves garlic, minced
- ❖ 1 tablespoon grated fresh ginger
- ❖ 1 teaspoon sesame oil
- ❖ 1/4 teaspoon red pepper flakes
- ❖ 1/4 cup chopped peanuts (for garnish)
- ❖ Chopped fresh cilantro (for garnish)
- ❖ Cooked rice or noodles for serving

INSTRUCTIONS:

1. In the slow cooker, add bite-sized chicken breasts, thinly sliced onions, bell peppers, chicken broth, creamy peanut butter, soy sauce, honey, rice vinegar, chopped garlic, grated fresh ginger, sesame oil, and red pepper flakes. Mix everything.
2. simmer: Cover and simmer chicken on low for 6–8 hours or high for 3–4 hours until soft and done.
3. Cornstarch slurry can thicken the sauce. Stir 1 tablespoon cornstarch and 2 teaspoons water in a small bowl until

smooth. Add cornstarch slurry to slow cooker in last 30 minutes. Stir the sauce and let it thicken.

4. Heat Thai Peanut Chicken and serve over noodles or rice. For garnish, chop fresh cilantro and peanuts.

NOTE:

- ➢ Chicken: Use boneless, skinless breasts for this recipe. You can also use chicken thighs.
- ➢ Peanut Butter: Creamy peanut butter enriches the rich sauce. Use creamy or natural peanut butter.
- ➢ Reduce meal salt with low-sodium soy sauce.
- ➢ Honey: Adjust sweetness to your liking.
- ➢ Use more or fewer red pepper flakes depending on your heat tolerance.
- ➢ Fresh cilantro and chopped peanuts provide crunch to the dish. Add lime juice or green onion slices if desired.
- ➢ Leftover Thai peanut chicken can be refrigerated in an airtight container for three days. Reheat gently in the microwave or stove before serving.

INGREDIENTS:

- ❖ 2 cans (15 oz each) of chickpeas (garbanzo beans), drained and rinsed
- ❖ 1 onion, diced
- ❖ 2 cloves garlic, minced
- ❖ 2 carrots, diced
- ❖ 2 celery stalks, diced
- ❖ 1 bell pepper, diced (any color)
- ❖ 1 can (14.5 oz) diced tomatoes, undrained
- ❖ 3 cups vegetable broth or chicken broth
- ❖ 1 teaspoon smoked paprika
- ❖ 1 teaspoon ground cumin
- ❖ 1/2 teaspoon dried thyme
- ❖ 1/2 teaspoon dried oregano
- ❖ Salt and pepper to taste
- ❖ 2 cups chopped spinach or kale
- ❖ Chopped fresh parsley or cilantro for garnish
- ❖ Crusty bread for serving

INSTRUCTIONS:

1. Diced tomatoes, onion, celery, carrots, bell pepper, ground cumin, smoked paprika, dried thyme, dried oregano, salt, and pepper should be added to the slow cooker. Mix everything.
2. Cover and cook vegetables for 6-8 hours on low or 3-4 hours on high to soften.
3. Add Greens: Stir in chopped spinach or kale 30 minutes before serving to wilt.

Serve:

- Ladle hot Spanish Chickpea Stew into bowls and top with chopped cilantro or parsley. Serve on the side or with fresh bread for dipping.

NOTES:

- ➤ Chickpeas: If desired, dried or canned garbanzo beans can be substituted for the canned version in this recipe. Drain and rinse them before placing them in the slow cooker.
- ➤ vegetables: Chopped bell pepper, celery, carrots, onions, and garlic provide the stew's taste and texture. You are welcome to include other veggies, such as chopped butternut squash, zucchini, or potatoes.
- ➤ Broth: For a non-vegetarian alternative, use chicken broth; for a vegetarian variant, use vegetable broth. The broth enhances the stew's flavor.
- ➤ Spices: The stew's distinctive Spanish taste comes from adding smoked paprika, ground cumin, dried thyme, and dried oregano. Adapt the quantity of spices to your personal inclinations.
- ➤ Greens: Chopped kale or spinach adds more nutrients and a fresh taste to the stew. You can also use collard greens, chard, or any other leafy green.
- ➤ Garnish: Finely chopped cilantro or parsley gives the meal a fresh flavor. To taste, you can garnish with a little lemon juice or extra virgin olive oil.
- ➤ You may store any leftover Spanish Chickpea Stew in the fridge for up to three days if you seal it properly. Return to a moderate simmer over low heat until ready to serve.

INGREDIENTS:

- ❖ 1.5 pounds of skinless, boneless chicken thighs
- ❖ one-fourth cup of honey
- ❖ 1/4 cup soy sauce
- ❖ 3 cloves garlic, minced
- ❖ 1 tablespoon rice vinegar
- ❖ 1 tablespoon sesame oil
- ❖ 1 tablespoon cornstarch (optional for thickening)
- ❖ 1 tablespoon water (optional for thickening)
- ❖ Sesame seeds, for garnish
- ❖ Chopped green onions for garnish
- ❖ Cooked rice for serving

INSTRUCTIONS:

1. Mixing Ingredients in Slow Cooker: In the slow cooker, thoroughly whisk together the rice vinegar, sesame oil, honey, soy sauce, and minced garlic. After adding them to the slow cooker, turn the skinless, boneless chicken thighs to coat them with sauce.
2. Cook:
3. Simmer, covered, for 6-8 hours on low heat or 3-4 hours on high heat, or until chicken is absolutely tender.
4. A cornstower slurry will help you thicken the sauce. In a small bowl, mix one tablespoon water and one tablespoon cornstarch until thick. In last 30 minutes of simmering, stir cornstarch slurry into slow cooker. Stirring often helps to thicken the sauce.

Serve:

- Place the warmed Honey Garlic Chicken on top of the prepared rice. Give chopped green onions and sesame seeds as garnishes to give more crunch and taste.

NOTES:

➢ For this dish, skinless, boneless chicken thighs are best because they retain their moisture and tenderness well when cooked slowly. But you may also use chicken breasts.

➢ Honey: Use pure honey for the most flavor. Adjust the amount of honey to get the right sweetness.

➢ To make the dish less salty, use soy sauce with low sodium.

➢ Garlic: The chicken gains a fragrant flavor from freshly minced garlic. You can change the amount of garlic to suit your tastes.

➢ Rice Vinegar: Rice vinegar adds a small acidity to counterbalance the honey's sweetness. If necessary, you can substitute apple cider vinegar.

➢ Thickness: The cornstarch slurry makes the sauce shinier and more dense. If you would like a thinner sauce, you can skip this step.

➢ Garnishes: Chopped green onions and sesame seeds give the meal more taste and visual appeal. For added spiciness, garnish with sliced red chili peppers.

➢ Storage: You may store any excess honey garlic chicken for up to three days in the fridge if you seal it tightly. Warm it up a little in the oven or microwave before serving.

INGREDIENTS:

- ❖ 1 pound Italian sausage, casings removed
- ❖ 1 onion, diced
- ❖ 2 cloves garlic, minced
- ❖ 2 carrots, diced
- ❖ 2 celery stalks, diced
- ❖ 1 bell pepper, diced (any color)
- ❖ 1 can (14.5 oz) diced tomatoes, undrained
- ❖ 4 cups chicken broth
- ❖ 1 teaspoon dried basil
- ❖ 1 teaspoon dried oregano
- ❖ 1/2 teaspoon dried thyme
- ❖ Salt and pepper to taste
- ❖ 2 cups chopped spinach or kale
- ❖ 1 cup small pasta
- ❖ Grated Parmesan cheese for serving
- ❖ Crusty bread for serving

INSTRUCTIONS:

1. Prepare the Italian sausage by breaking it up with a spoon and browning it in a skillet over medium heat. Pour off any surplus fat if necessary.
2. Fill the slow cooker with all the ingredients. Place the cooked Italian sausage into the slow cooker. Add the diced tomatoes and their liquids, chopped onion, minced garlic, celery, carrots, and bell pepper. Add the dried thyme, basil, oregano, salt, pepper, and chicken stock. Combine all of the ingredients.

3. Cook: Cover and boil the vegetables for 6–8 hours on low or 3–4 hours on high or until tender.
4. Add the greens and pasta: About 30 minutes before serving, toss in the raw spaghetti and chopped kale or spinach. Cook the pasta until it's al dente, covered.

Serve hot Italian sausage soup with grated Parmesan cheese on top. Serve with toasted bread on the side.

NOTES:

> Use spicy or mild Italian sausage; the choice is yours. Use turkey-based Italian sausage instead for a lighter alternative.
> Dietary vegetables: The soup gets its taste and texture from chopped carrots, celery, onion, and garlic. Feel free to incorporate more veggies such diced potatoes, zucchini, or cannellini beans.
> Tomatoes: Chopped tomatoes from a can provide a substantial base for the soup. You can get extra flavor by roasting diced tomatoes over a fire.
> Broth: Use chicken broth to make a flavorful base. You can substitute low-sodium chicken broth if you prefer.
> Herbs: The soup has a classic Italian flavor thanks to the dried basil, oregano, and thyme. You can also add fresh herbs if they are available.
> Greens: Chopped spinach or kale adds additional nutrition to the soup. Any other leafy green, such as escarole or Swiss chard, can also be used.

- ➢ Pasta: Elbow macaroni, ditalini, or tiny shells are suitable small pasta shapes for this soup. Adjust the cooking time as recommended on the pasta's package.
- ➢ Garnish: A last, savory touch to the soup is a grating of Parmesan cheese. For garnish, try a little extra virgin olive oil or fresh, freshly chopped parsley.
- ➢ Refrigerate any remaining Italian sausage soup in an airtight container for up to three days. Before serving, gently reheat over low heat.

INGREDIENTS:

- ❖ 1 pound boneless, skinless chicken breasts
- ❖ 4 cups chicken broth
- ❖ 4 cups frozen corn kernels
- ❖ 2 potatoes, peeled and diced
- ❖ 1 onion, diced
- ❖ 2 cloves garlic, minced
- ❖ 2 carrots, diced
- ❖ 2 celery stalks, diced
- ❖ 1 bell pepper, diced (any color)
- ❖ 1 can (14.5 oz) diced tomatoes, undrained
- ❖ 1 teaspoon dried thyme
- ❖ 1 teaspoon dried parsley
- ❖ 1/2 teaspoon paprika
- ❖ 1/2 teaspoon dried rosemary
- ❖ Salt and pepper to taste
- ❖ 1 cup heavy cream or half-and-half
- ❖ 2 tablespoons all-purpose flour
- ❖ Chopped fresh parsley for garnish
- ❖ Cooked and crumbled bacon for garnish (optional)

INSTRUCTIONS:

1. Place skinless, boneless chicken breasts in slow cooker. Combine ingredients. Add chicken stock, frozen corn kernels, chopped celery, sliced carrots, diced onion, minced garlic, dried thyme, parsley, paprika, rosemary, diced tomatoes (with liquids), and salt and pepper. Mix everything.
2. Simmer: Simmer, covered, for 6-8 hours on low heat or 3-4 hours on high heat, until chicken and veggies are tender.
3. Shred Chicken: Remove slow-cooked chicken breasts and shred with two forks. Put the chicken shreds back in the slow cooker.
4. Whisk heavy cream (or half-and-half) and all-purpose flour in a small bowl to thicken the chowder. Stir cream mixture in slow cooker until mixed. The chowder will thicken after 30 more minutes on high with a lid.

Serve

- Chicken and Corn Chowder in dishes, topping with cooked and crumbled bacon (if desired).

NOTE:

- ➤ Although thighs would work just as well, this recipe asks for skinless, boneless chicken breasts.
- ➤ Chopped bell pepper, celery, carrots, onions, and garlic give the chowder flavor and texture. You can add diced zucchini or potatoes.
- ➤ The chowder's sweetness and texture originate from frozen corn kernels. You can use fresh corn kernels if available.
- ➤ Broth: Chicken broth underpins chowder. Low-sodium chicken broth is another option.
- ➤ Spices and herbs: Dried thyme, parsley, paprika, and rosemary flavor the chowder. Adjust the seasoning to your liking.
- ➤ Heavy cream or half-and-half adds creaminess to chowder. Whole milk is lighter.
- ➤ Thickening: Mix half-and-half or heavy cream and all-purpose flour to thicken soup. Skip this step for thinner chowder.
- ➤ Chowder garnishes: Crumbled bacon and minced fresh parsley add color and taste. Garnish with cheese crumbs or chopped green onions if you choose.
- ➤ Storage: Refrigerate leftover chicken and corn chowder for three days in an airtight container. Reheat slowly on the burner before serving.

INGREDIENTS:

- ❖ 1 cup rinsed, drained, dried red lentils
- ❖ 1 onion, diced
- ❖ 3 cloves garlic, minced
- ❖ 1 tablespoon grated fresh ginger
- ❖ 1 bell pepper, diced (any color)
- ❖ 1 carrot, diced
- ❖ 1 can (14.5 oz) diced tomatoes, undrained
- ❖ 1 can (13.5 oz) coconut milk
- ❖ 2 cups vegetable broth or chicken broth
- ❖ 2 tablespoons curry powder
- ❖ 1 teaspoon ground cumin
- ❖ 1 teaspoon ground turmeric
- ❖ 1/2 teaspoon ground coriander
- ❖ 1/4 teaspoon cayenne pepper (optional for heat)
- ❖ Salt and pepper to taste
- ❖ Juice of 1 lime
- ❖ Chopped fresh cilantro for garnish
- ❖ Cooked rice or naan bread for serving

INSTRUCTIONS:

1. The ingredients to be combined in the slow cooker are rinsed red lentils, diced onion, minced garlic, grated fresh ginger, diced bell pepper, diced carrot, diced tomatoes (with their juices), diced turmeric, diced coriander, diced cumin, curry powder, ground cumin, ground coriander, and cayenne pepper (if using), along with coconut milk and vegetable or chicken broth. Mix everything.

2. Simmer: Cover and cook for 6–8 hours on low or 3–4 hours on high until lentils are mushy and flavors have integrated.
3. Season the curry with extra curry powder, spices, salt, and pepper to taste.
4. Finish: To lighten the taste, stir in the lime juice before serving.

Serve:

- Top the hot Red Lentil Curry with freshly chopped cilantro. For a full dinner, serve with naan bread or boiled rice.

NOTES:

- ➤ Red Lentils: This recipe calls for dried red lentils. Rinse and drain them before placing them in the slow cooker.
- ➤ Vegetables: Diced onion, garlic, bell pepper, and carrot enhance curry's flavor and texture. Add more veggies like spinach, chopped potatoes, or cauliflower florets.
- ➤ Tomatoes: The curry's acidity and rich taste come from canned chopped tomatoes. Diced tomatoes roasted over a fire can provide more flavor.
- ➤ Coconut Milk: Full-fat coconut milk makes rich, creamy dishes. Half the coconut milk makes the curry lighter, but it may need additional creaminess.
- ➤ Spices: The curry's fragrant flavor and warmth come from curry powder, ground cumin, ground turmeric, ground coriander, and cayenne pepper if used. Adapt the quantity of spices to your inclinations.

- ➤ Garnish: Chopped fresh cilantro gives the curry's final dish a vibrant flavor. You may add a dollop of yogurt or some sliced red chile peppers to the top.
- ➤ Storage: KeepYou may store any leftover red lentil curry in the fridge for up to three days if you seal it well. Return to a moderate simmer over low heat until ready to serve.

Conclusion

In conclusion, slow-cooking cookbooks are an excellent tool for streamlining meal planning and elevating the dining experience.They have a ton of delicious and simple recipes. These cookbooks are excellent for both novice and experienced cooks due to their diverse selection of dishes that cater to various palates and dietary needs. For home cooks, slow cooking is a great method to save time and energy without sacrificing flavor or texture. The hands-off cooking approach makes meal preparation a breeze, which is ideal for families or individuals with demanding schedules. With just a few key ingredients and slow cooking, you can create delectable dishes that will please even the pickiest palates.

In addition, slow-cooking textbooks frequently showcase an array of flavors and cuisines, enabling cooks to try out new dishes and broaden their culinary experiences. There's bound to be a slow-cooking dish that suits your mood, be it for tender braised meats, rich sweets, or hearty stews and soups.

Additionally, there are lots of helpful tips in slow-cooking cookbooks if you want to know how to get the most out of your slow cooker. These cookbooks are indispensable for consistently preparing flawlessly cooked meals.They go over everything, including understanding cooking times and temperatures and choosing the appropriate size and model. Furthermore, they typically include ideas for adjusting recipes to suit individual preferences or dietary restrictions, ensuring that slow cooking is within reach of everybody.

All things considered, slow-cooking cookbooks are an invaluable tool for anyone wishing to streamline the cooking process, increase their culinary skills, or savor tasty, home-cooked meals with little work. These cookbooks will become a useful tool in any kitchen because to their delicious food, simple-to-follow instructions, and helpful hints. Hence, a slow-cooking cookbook is an indispensable addition to your kitchen library, regardless of your level of experience—whether you're a seasoned chef trying to shake things up or a novice excited to dive into the realm of slow cooking.

THE END

Made in the USA
Columbia, SC
24 September 2024

42731007R00139